ABBOT'S HOSPITAL GUILDFORD

Brian Taylor

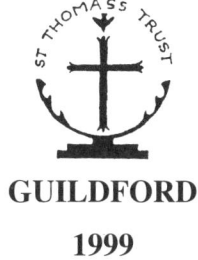

GUILDFORD
1999

ABBOT'S HOSPITAL GUILDFORD

First published in Great Britain 1999

© St Thomas's Trust

All rights reserved. No part of this book may be reproduced in any form by any means, electronic or mechanical, including photocopying, recording or by any information system, without permission in writing from the publisher.

British Library cataloguing in Publication Data. A catalogue record for this book will be available from the British Library.

Published by St Thomas's Trust,
Vine Cottage, Sutton Park, Guildford GU4 7QN.

Printed by Biddles Ltd, Guildford and King's Lynn

ISBN 0 9520140 4 1

CONTENTS

Foreword v
List of Illustrations vi
Preface vii

Chapter 1	– The Founder and his Family	1
Chapter 2	– The Foundation	19
Chapter 3	– The Manufacture and the School	33
Chapter 4	– The Hospital 1633 - 1846	45
Chapter 5	– The Reformed Community	69
Chapter 6	– Modern Times	107
Appendix 1	– The Masters of the Hospital	119
Appendix 2	– The First Statutes	123
Appendix 3	– The Victorian Statutes	147
Appendix 4	– Book List	155
Index		159

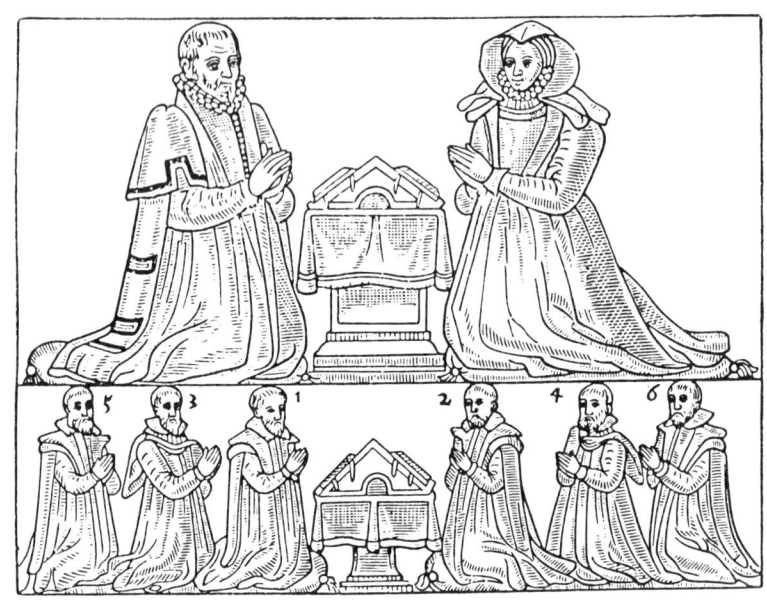

HERE LIE THE BODIES OF MAVRICE ABBOT & ALICE HIS WIFE, INHABITANTS OF THIS TOWNE OF GVILD= FORD, WHO LIVED TOGETHER MARIED 58. YEARES. & HAD. 6. SONES ALL WHOME THEY LEFT ALIVE. SHEE DYED THE. 15. OF SEPTEMBER. 1606. BEING. 80. YEERE OLD AND HE THE. 25.TH OF THE SAME, MO+ NETH AND YEERE: BEING OF AGE. 86. YEERES. BOTH IN ASSVRED HOPE OF A IOYFVLL RESVRREC=TION.

The memorial plate to Maurice and Alice Abbot in Holy Trinity Church. Their six sons were Anthony (Mayor of Guildford in 1598), Richard (first Master of the hospital), Robert (Bishop of Salisbury), George (its founder), Maurice (Lord Mayor of London) and John.

The brass in Holy Trinity Church
George Abbot is number 4

FOREWORD

Brian Taylor was inducted into the Guildford parish of St Nicolas in 1975 and resigned the living in 1993.

During his time as Rector he was *ex officio* a Governor of the Hospital of the Blessed Trinity, known colloquially as Abbot's Hospital. He was assiduous in his duties as Governor and his advice, always succinct and to the point, was welcomed by his colleagues during their deliberations.

His devotion to this ancient "house of pity" led him, at the request of his fellow Governors, to undertake the immense task of writing what is surely a definitive history of the place from its beginning, early in the seventeenth century, until the present day. This has been a labour of pure love. He has produced a work of painstaking and meticulous scholarship which merits our gratitude and praise.

As the next millennium approaches, what does the future hold for Abbot's Hospital?

It would be bold, even unwise, to speculate, but what is fairly certain is that the year 2000 AD will see an ageing population throughout the whole of the developed world. The elderly will have rising expectations in such matters as pensions, accommodation, health care and generally as to the quality of their lives. It is to be hoped that, in its turn, society will recognise that older people with their long experience of life can make a valuable contribution to the wider community.

The Hospital is well placed to meet the likely requirements of the immediate future. The accommodation which it provides is comfortable; the health of its residents is its first concern, and its central position in Guildford High Street enables them to mix with the outside world as much as or as little as they wish. And indeed, with due regard to their privacy, the outside world is frequently present within the Hospital's walls as guided tours are conducted rounds its premises.

If, as many fear, the prevailing collective neurosis of western society is meaninglessness, then the chapel of the Hospital will continue to provide solace and assurance for many of the residents. Its services, which are frequent and well attended, remind the congregation that there is a dimension to life which is outside time, that eternal values are in the end the only ones worth striving for, and that underneath the flux of our temporal existence are the everlasting arms.

June 1995   JOHN BROWN
                                                 Chairman of the Board of Governors

ILLUSTRATIONS
between pages 88 and 89

Frontispiece – The brass in Holy Trinity Church

1. The courtyard, drawn by Alexander Munro, 4 September 1837 (Guildford Museum)
2. The House of Industry, drawn by John Hassell in 1822
3. The High Street front, drawn by G.S.Shepherd for E.W.Brayley's *A Topical History of Surrey*, London 1841
4. The chapel, drawn by J.R.Thompson for Brayley
5. The hall, drawn by J.R.Thompson for Brayley
6. The Hospital gateway c 1865, from a photograph by J.Chaplin (Eric Hunter)
7. The Hospital seal
8. The fire of 1916 (from the Guildford Remembrancer, volume 1; Surrey Local Studies Library)
9. The Governors' meeting on 29 November 1984, photograph by John Hyde-Smith
10. The new courtyard, photograph by H.G.Taylor

    Cover design by Tollard Royal, using a photograph by John Hyde-Smith

PREFACE

In sixteenth century England, monastic houses and chantries gave place to schools, colleges and houses for the aged poor as a way of perpetuating benefactors' names and shewing gratitude for accumulated wealth. Abbot's Hospital, as it is usually called, takes its place among these, founded by a bachelor Archbishop of Canterbury in his native town in the reign of James I.

Sometimes the events which stirred the nation affected the lives of those who lived in the hospital, but more often they were disturbed or enlivened by things that happened closer at hand. These will both take their place in this story, but its main purpose is to record the development of the life of a group of elderly men and women in the centre of their own town. Attention will also be given to the endowment of the hospital, and the ways in which income and expenditure have been balanced through the centuries, not always successfully. A separate account is given of George Abbot's other foundation in Guildford, the "manufacture", intended to assist those engaged in making cloth, and its later development as a school.

Soon after I became Rector of St Nicolas' in 1975, I became aware that I was an official Governor of Trinity Hospital - but I received no word from it. After a while I called, and shortly after that I had a letter from R.H. Percy, the clerk to the Governors, which began,

> As you probably know the Rector of St. Nicholas is an Ex-officio Governor of this Hospital. No Rector of St.Nicholas has attended any of the meetings of functions at this Hospital for some years past, but I hope very much that you will be able to visit us here from time to time, even though you may not be able to attend the monthly meetings regularly.

and he ended,

> I would be grateful if you would let me know whether you will be able to attend the Hospital functions, in which case I will send you the monthly notices and Minutes etc.

I attended my first meeting on 30 October, and from then until my resignation from St Nicolas' in 1993 I was rarely absent. We all have to make our scales of priorities, and the immediate interest that the hospital aroused ensured that I could always find time for the Governors' meetings, and to take an active part in their business.

These have been very exciting years. In 1975 life in the hospital was not much different from what it had been in the early seventeenth century. The brothers and sisters lived in single rooms, with very little comfort or convenience. Now they have flats or houses, and the community includes married couples - whether the Founder would like it or not.

His main intentions, however, are honoured; homes and security are provided for needy citizens of his native town.

The records of the hospital are almost complete, and are kept, as the Founder directed, in the upper room of the gatehouse. Some of the documents relating to the original endowment farms are from as early as the fourteenth century. This valuable archive has been the main source for the research for this book. Assistance came in an unexpected way. Philip Palmer, who was master from 1913 to 1926, spent much of his spare time reading the hospital records. In 1918 he began to make transcripts and notes, and filled five large volumes, covering the years 1614 to 1861. At the beginning of the first book he wrote, "To be kept in custody of Surrey Archaeological Society, but not used until used as a whole by a competent person". Subsequently the Society's name was deleted and "Lambeth Library" written above. I am grateful to the Library Committee at Lambeth Palace for reckoning me a competent person, and for allowing the volumes to be kept in the Guildford Muniment Room while I worked through them. They are more than transcripts, for Palmer often points the way to conclusions, which can be tested, and refers to material other than hospital records. (Lambeth Palace Library MSS 1410-1414)

I have received willing help from the staff of Lambeth Palace Library, the Guildford Muniment Room and of the Local Studies Library in Guildford. Those who have assisted me with information about particular points are acknowledged in the notes. For recent years, masters of the hospital, clerks to the Governors and their secretary have helped me to give an accurate account. Permission to use illustrations is recorded in the list, and I thank those who have provided them. Most of all I am grateful to my fellow Governors who, as long ago as 1984 encouraged me to write this book, and gave me permission to use the hospital records.

BRIAN TAYLOR

ONE
THE FOUNDER AND HIS FAMILY

The Abbots were a Suffolk family, and lived at Chelsworth as early as 1260.[1] Thomas Abbot, the Archbishop's grandfather, was a clothworker. He was a younger son, and moved from Chelsworth to Hawkedon. His son Maurice, also a clothworker, lived for a while in Farnham, and moved to Guildford before or after his marriage to Alice Marsh, which took place in St Mary's Guildford on 30 June 1548. The English reformation was still in its early stages, and its direction was not then sure.

The repudiation of papal authority in England was completed in 1534. Bishop John Fisher and Sir Thomas More were executed in 1535, and Thomas Cromwell in 1540. Thomas Cranmer, twice married and the father of at least two children, had been Archbishop of Canterbury since 1532, but the Bishop of Winchester, in whose diocese Guildford lay, had since 1531 been the catholic-minded Stephen Gardiner. The placing of the English Bible in every parish church was ordered in 1536, the year that the general dissolution of the monasteries and other religious houses began. The Dominican friary in Guildford was surrendered on 10 October 1538. King Edward VI ascended the throne on 28 January 1547, with Edward Seymour Duke of Somerset as protector until 1549. Soon, in 1547, chantry foundations were abolished. Maurice Abbot and Alice Marsh probably received Holy Communion in both kinds for the first time at Easter 1548, but for their wedding three months later the Latin rite of the Sarum manual would be used. The first son of the marriage, Richard, born in 1549, may have had a Latin rite baptism, or perhaps was born after the issue of the first Edwardian prayer book. The second son, Anthony,[2] probably was baptized with the form in either the 1549 or 1552 prayer book, Robert (1560), George (1562), Morris[3] (1565) and John (1567) were all born after the publication of the 1559 prayer book of Elizabeth I.

Daniel Featley, one of George Abbot's chaplains, writing about Robert Abbot, said that "his Parents embraced the truth of the Gospell in King *Edwards* dayes, and were persecuted for it in Queen *Maries* raigne (by Doctor *Story* of infamous memory) and not-withstanding all troubles and molestations continued constant in the profession of the truth till their death, and all their children treading in their holy steps, *walked with a right foot to the Gospell*, and were zealous professors of the reformed Religion".[4] No details of this persecution are known. John Story, who changed sides twice, was Chancellor of the diocese of London for Bishop Edmund Bonner, and one of the most active agents of the Queen. He was executed for treason on 1 June 1571, when the future archbishop was eight, old enough to understand.[5]

Anthony Wood, in his records of Oxford men, preserved the information that at some time before the birth of their third son, Maurice and Alice moved across the Wey. There

Abbot's Hospital Guildford

Robert was born in 1560, and George on 29 October 1562, "in an House now an Alehouse, bearing the sign of the *Three Mariners*, by the River's side - near the Bridge, on the North side of the Street, in St. Nicholas's Parish".[6] George Abbot was baptized at St Nicolas' on 30 October. The rector at that time was William Saxey, who was sufficiently pliable to retain this and other benefices through all the changes from the last months of Henry VIII's reign until well into the reign of Elizabeth I. In 1562, it was said of him in reply to articles of enquiry from Archbishop Parker that he was nonresident, so it is unlikely that he baptized the future archbishop. The family moved back across the river to Holy Trinity parish, where the two youngest sons were baptized, Morris in 1565 and John in 1567.

The rectory of Holy Trinity was vacant from 1562 to 1593, and it is therefore not possible to know who was responsible for Church influence on the Abbot brothers as they grew up. Two curates were also masters of the Grammar School, Roger Goad in the fifteen-sixties, whose son Thomas was later to be George's best-known chaplain, and Francis Taylor, 1575-1580. Both of these may have been assistant masters before their appointment as head.[7] Robert, George and Morris are known to have attended the school. George remembered Taylor, and shewed his appreciation by appointing him Vicar of Lambeth in 1611.

Only Robert and George went to the university. Robert entered Balliol College Oxford in 1575, and matriculated on 26 December 1577. George followed him to the same college in 1578, and matriculated on 2 May 1581.[8] Richard, Anthony and John remained in Guildford, where their sorrows and joys are recorded in the registers of Holy Trinity and St Mary's. Anthony was mayor in 1598. John practised law as an attorney. Morris sought prosperity in London, and succeeded, as a woollen draper and merchant. He was one of the original directors of the East India Company when it received its charter in 1600, and became a governor in 1624. In that year he also became a member of the council of the Virginia Company. He was elected to Parliament for Kingston-upon-Hull in 1621 and 1624, and for the city of London in Charles I's first Parliament in 1625. In that year he was the first person to be knighted by King Charles after his accession. In the city of London he became an alderman in 1626, sheriff in 1627 and Lord Mayor in 1638. At the end of his year in that office he retired from public life, and died in 1642. The Archbishop admired success, and turned to Morris for advice and help with his charitable activities.

Abbot graduated as a bachelor of arts on 31 May 1582, and on 29 November 1583 he was elected a fellow of Balliol, joining his brother Robert in the fellowship. For several years they were together, becoming known as strong upholders of Calvinist theology, and opponents of any tendency or leniency towards Roman Catholicism. The dates of their ordination are not known. Their partnership was broken when Robert resigned his fellowship to become Rector of All Saints Worcester in 1589.

The Founder and His Family

George Abbot became a master of arts on 17 December 1585. He was appointed to several college offices, junior dean in 1587 and 1598, junior bursar in 1588 and 1590, senior dean in 1592, 1595 and 1596, and notary in 1597. Robert and George were admitted as bachelors of divinity on the same day, 4 March 1594. In that same year William Laud was elected a fellow of St. John's College. He very soon gained a reputation for maintaining the catholic tradition in the Church of England. This brought him into conflict with the Abbot brothers, and for George at least, the disapproval and dislike became obsessive, and aggravated by frequent contact for forty years, in the affairs of the university, the Church and the State. The background and early education of the two men - Laud was the son of a Reading clothworker, and educated at Reading School - were closely similar, and Laud's career followed a course very much like Abbot's. Merit and scholarship alone were not sufficient to win high office; access to influence and patronage was necessary. George Abbot was noticed by the puritan nobleman Thomas Sackville, Lord Buckhurst, who was Chancellor of the university from 1591 until his death in 1608.[9] Abbot became Sackville's chaplain, and later in the century began to receive his reward. On 6 September 1597 he was elected Master of University College, the fellows complying with the wish of the Chancellor. As the head of a college Abbot served as Vice-chancellor of the university three times, in 1600, 1603 and 1605. in the second of these turns he had the irritation of Laud, who was in office as junior proctor. The college grew in membership under his mastership, despite his strictness, and his measures against long hair, drinking, and other undergraduate excesses.

In 1600 Abbot received his first ecclesiastical appointment, when he was chosen by the Crown to be Dean of Winchester, and was installed on 6 March. It was said that he paid £600 for this preferment. There is no evidence that he spent much time in Winchester, but the deanery gave him a place in the convocation of Canterbury, and so brought him in closer touch with central Church authority, and with affairs in London.

When James I came to England in 1603, Abbot, as Vice-chancellor, met him for the first time. He went to Woodstock to greet the King on behalf of the university. At first it was Robert who won more royal favour. He became a chaplain to the King early in the reign, and was also approved by the protestant-minded Prince Henry, the elder son of the King.

George Abbot produced a number of books while he was in Oxford. In 1598 he published his thesis for the degree of doctor of divinity, which he took on 9 May 1597, *Quaestiones Sex*, a consideration of six propositions, dealt with on the basis of Calvinist theology.[10] In 1599 there followed *A Brief Description of the whole World*, written for students, and reprinted several times in Abbot's lifetime and afterwards.[11] A less popular book appeared in 1600, *An Exposition upon the Prophet Ionah*, thirty sermons preached on the book in St Mary's Oxford.[12] A major work of religious controversy was published in 1604, *The Reasons which Doctour Hill hath brought, for the upholding of Papistry, which is falselie termed the Catholike Religion: Unmasked, and Showed to be very weake, and upon examination most insufficient for that purpose.*[13] Thomas Hill, a convert to Roman Catholicism, had published *A Quartron of Reasons of Catholicke Religion* in 1600, and

Abbot's Hospital Guildford

Abbot's work is a point by point refuting of Hill's case. A little later Robert Abbot was engaged in a more prolonged controversy with a more important Roman Catholic, William Bishop, and published *A Defence of the Reformed Catholicke of Mr William Perkins, lately deceased, against the bastard Counter-Catholicke of Dr Bishop*, which appeared in parts from 1606 to 1609.[14] It was dedicated to Prince Henry, and brought Robert again into public notice. In 1609 he returned to Oxford as Master of Balliol, and also became Regius Professor of Divinity in 1612.

As King James travelled southwards through England after his accession, he was met by a puritan deputation, which presented the Millenary Petition, asking for changes in Church practice. James summoned a conference in an attempt to settle the disputes in the Church. It met at Hampton Court in January 1604. The puritans gained little, but the most important outcome of the conference was the decision to prepare a revised translation of the Bible. The task was divided among six companies, and Abbot was a member of one of those in Oxford. This company, under the direction of the Regius Professor of Greek, John Perin, translated the Gospels, the Acts of the Apostles, and Revelation.[15] The "Authorised Version" was published in 1611.

The Earl of Dorset, Thomas Sackville, died on 19 April 1608. George Abbot preached at the funeral in Westminster Abbey.[16] Dorset was succeeded as Chancellor of the university by Richard Bancroft, who had been Archbishop of Canterbury since 1604, and who was not likely to advance Abbot's interests. A new patron was found in George Home, Treasurer of Scotland since 1601, and a close friend and adviser of King James, who revived the earldom of Dunbar for him in 1605. Abbot became Dunbar's chaplain in 1608, and very soon was brought into public affairs.

After the Hampton Court Conference, and with the knowledge of the reforms that Bancroft was pursuing in the Church of England,[17] James decided to bring order into the Church in Scotland. During his reign as James VI, from 1567, he had suffered much from the power of Presbyterians, and he wished to re-establish episcopal government in the Church. In 1608 the thirteen dioceses had nominal bishops, lawfully provided, and drawing the revenues of their sees, but none had been consecrated, and the succession had been lost. In that year Dunbar was sent to Scotland, and Abbot was one of those who accompanied him. The King hoped that the English and Scottish Churches could be united, but this was more than the Scottish protestants could accept. Abbot won their sympathy by his own Calvinist convictions, and persuaded them that agreement to the consecration of bishops was not necessarily a weakening in the direction of prelacy and popery. King James readily approved the compromise, and it was accepted by the Parliament of Scotland. Abbot's part in this well exemplifies his attitude to Church government, and indeed to Church affairs generally. His insistence on proper order was based on a desire for orderliness and control, rather than a wish to uphold order in any catholic sense. It was later said that at one point in Scotland he had been inclined to give way to the Presbyterians, but others of the party warned Dunbar, who made sure that the King's wishes were not drastically reduced.[18]

The Founder and His Family

In 1609 Abbot received a further reward. On 9 April William Overton, Bishop of Coventry and Lichfield, died. George Abbot was nominated to succeed him, and was elected by the chapter on 27 May. For some reason the election was not confirmed until 2 December. He was consecrated at Lambeth on 3 December by Archbishop Bancroft, assisted by Lancelot Andrewes of Ely and Richard Neile of Rochester.[19] At that time his diocese included Staffordshire and Derbyshire, most of Warwickshire and much of Shropshire. He approached his work without any experience of parochial or pastoral ministry; unlike his brother Robert - and also unlike William Laud a little later, he had never left the university to look after a parish. In his favour it should be said that unlike many of his contemporaries, he had never accumulated benefices and dignities, with the one exception of the deanery of Winchester, which he resigned soon after he was nominated as bishop. There are no records of Abbot's Lichfield episcopate; indeed there can have been little to record. Thomas Ravis, Bishop of London since 1607, died on 14 December. Abbot was nominated to succeed him on 24 December - exactly three weeks after his consecration to Lichfield. His election was confirmed on 20 January, and he was enthroned on 12 February. On 23 February he resigned his mastership of University College Oxford.

The bishop took his seat in the House of Lords on 9 February 1610, and became a regular attender, and a member of several committees. Later in the year, in November, he became a member of the Inner Temple. Now that he had no responsibilities in Oxford, he was able to be very active in his diocese, which at that time included Middlesex and Essex and the southern half of Hertfordshire, as well as the city of London. It was while he was Bishop of London that Abbot was asked to complete what had been agreed for the Scottish Church. Three of the nominal bishops were sent to England for consecration, Gavin Hamilton of Galloway, Andrew Lamb of Brechin, and John Spottiswoode of Glasgow. Spottiswoode objected that if they received consecration from the Primate of All England, it would appear that they accepted that they were subject to the English Church. King James had already arranged that Abbot should preside over the consecration. It took place, with the assistance of Lancelot Andrewes of Ely and James Montague of Bath, on 21 October at London House. The three new bishops returned to Scotland, and by early May 1611 all the dioceses had consecrated bishops.[20]

Richard Bancroft, Archbishop of Canterbury, died on 2 November 1610. Most of the bishops hoped that he would be succeeded by Lancelot Andrewes of Ely. Thomas Bilson of Winchester and James Montague of Bath and Wells were also spoken of, but the Earl of Dunbar urged the King to appoint George Abbot. Dunbar died on 20 January 1611, but after an anxious pause, Abbot was nominated on 4 March. His election by the chapter of Canterbury on 18 March was confirmed on 9 April, and he was enthroned by proxy on 16 May. It was an unusually long primacy, twenty-two years and four months.[21] During that time there were new bishops in every diocese in England, except Sodor and Man. Two, Bath and Wells and Carlisle, had five changes, and several had four.

As Primate of All England, Abbot, who had been relatively unknown not many months before, became a prominent figure in the affairs of the nation. In April 1611 he joined the Court of High Commission, and in June he became a Privy Councillor, and he was present at most of the meetings. Later, in July 1618, he was made First Lord of the Treasury, when the Earl of Suffolk, the Lord High Treasurer, was suspended for embezzlement. Abbot held this position for over two years. In this summary of George Abbot's life, it is not possible to cover every aspect of his career. Instead a selection will be made of topics that reveal his character and interests. Political matters will be dealt with only incidentally.

The impression of George Abbot and his place in history that has prevailed was laid down by Edward Hyde, writing at the beginning of the eighteenth century. His opinion was that Abbot "had sat too many years in that See, and had too great Jurisdiction over the Church, though he was without any Credit in the Court from the death of King *James*, and had not much in many years before... He was a man of very morose manners, and a very sour aspect, which, in that time, was called Gravity... [He] was in truth totally ignorant of the true Constitution of the Church of *England*, and the State and Interest of the Clergy; as sufficiently appear'd through out the whole course of his life afterward."[22] Abbot's theological convictions were more in accord with lay opinion than were those of his opponents, but he came too late to enjoy power and influence for long. Changes in the royal circle were soon to leave him in a position of resentful reaction, and his inflexibility reduced his favour with the King.

The Archbishop considered that he had been raised up to promote and maintain the sort of protestantism that he had learnt in the middle years of Queen Elizabeth's reign, and intended to enforce right belief and right conduct. The Church of England, he thought, should unite the realm, and all protestants should be content to find in it what they needed. Abbot therefore opposed separatism, but also would deprive those who were flagrantly disloyal to Church practice. Foreign orders were recognized, and some Reformed ministers found benefices without episcopal ordination. He very quickly brought about a strengthening of the powers of the Commissioners Ecclesiastical, now to be called the High Commission, which had the authority of a court of law.[23] This was resented by the senior lawyers, and later led to increased unpopularity of the Church, especially when Laud succeeded to Canterbury. Early in Abbot's years as Archbishop, he was involved in the trial of two men for heresy, and supported the King in his determination that they should die if found guilty, as a sign of the orthodox intentions of the government. Bartholomew Legate was condemned, after standing firm against the personal persuasion of the King, for denying the divinity of Christ, and was burnt at Smithfield on 18 March 1612. Edward Wightman was burnt at Lichfield on 11 April in the same year, for denying the doctrine of the Trinity, and for claiming to be the Messiah and the Paraclete. They were the last to be executed for heresy in England. James led a change of feeling, that death should be replaced with solitary confinement as the penalty.

It was otherwise with Roman Catholics, against whom there was strong sentiment in the country; memories of the Armada were still fresh. James, the son of a Roman Catholic queen, wished to be lenient to loyal Roman Catholic laymen, but it was not possible to be tolerant to priests, or to converts, whose loyalty was necessarily doubtful. The Pope's claim to be able to depose rulers, and to release subjects from their allegiance, could not be accepted,for obvious political reasons.[24] The conflict was mismatched, for what seemed to one party to be accusation and execution for treachery, to the other was persecution and martyrdom for faith. Four Roman Catholics were killed in England in Abbot's brief London episcopate, and reckoned as martyrs, and twelve while he was Archbishop. The last of these was in 1628.[25] There then followed an interval until 1641 after Laud had been committed to the Tower of London.

At the beginning of the reign of King James, Abbot and those who followed him set their hopes on Prince Henry, the heir to the throne. As well as inheriting his mother's extravagance,[26] Henry was a convinced protestant, who hoped when he became king to bring back all the puritan separatists into the state Church. He was made Prince of Wales in June 1610, but died of typhoid on 6 November 1612, attended to the end by the Archbishop. This death was a turning point in English history - more than is often remembered, for in Henry's "grave were buried the hopes of the Puritan party.[27] Abbot understood that the future for protestantism was now less assured, with the eleven-year old Charles as heir. For the Archbishop the Princess Elizabeth became more important. He had supported her wedding with Frederic V, the Elector Palatine, and this took place early in 1613. He hoped that it would promote the interests of protestantism in Europe. Abbot's support for the King in allowing this match was far-sighted, for a grandson of the marriage was to become King, as George I, in 1714.

A less likely friendship existed between Abbot and James's Queen, Anne of Denmark, despite the uncertainty of her religious beliefs and allegiance. She supported Abbot when his influence began to decline, and her death on 2 March 1619 was a serious blow to him. Earlier she had tried to dissuade Abbot from helping George Villiers (later Earl, then Marquess, then Duke of Buckingham) to rise in the King's favour. The Archbishop thought that he would be a useful ally in the cause of protestantism, but the Queen rightly foresaw that Abbot would regret his choice.

This is not the place for a detailed account of English foreign relations in early Stuart times. For Abbot, religious considerations came first, and he found it hard to accept that political advantage should ever take precedence. James had hoped to ensure peace with Spain by bringing about the marriage of Prince Henry with a Spanish princess. The Prince was not at first compliant, but Abbot was reproved by the King for expressing dissent. Later the idea was revived for Prince Charles, but it came to nothing, to Abbot's relief.[28]

In August 1619, the Elector Frederic accepted the invitation of the people of Bohemia to become their king. Abbot encouraged this, to further the cause of protestantism in Europe, but he could not persuade King James or the Council. Germany and Spain invaded Bohemia, and defeated Frederic at the battle of the White Mountain, in November 1620. Frederic and Elizabeth, the "Winter Queen", were driven from the country. They lost the Palatinate too, and their life in exile began. James, influenced by Buckingham, and still with hopes of a Spanish marriage for Prince Charles, did not recognise his son-in-law as King, and did not go to his help.

James and the Archbishop were in agreement over the doctrinal controversy in Holland, between the Calvinists and the Arminians, who asserted the importance of free will, and the availability of saving grace to all men, against the determinist predestination upheld by the Calvinists. Quite apart from the theological principle, the King feared that the united protestant opposition to Rome could be weakened. The Calvinists summoned a synod at Dort, in 1618, at which the English Church was represented. The English delegates, who included Abbot's chaplain, Thomas Goad, signed the doctrinal articles condemning Arminianism, but affirmed the Church of England's retention of episcopacy.

Two other episodes illustrate Abbot's interest in the wider Church, as he found allies in his opposition to Rome. Kyrillos Loukaris was orthodox Patriarch of Alexandria when he began to look for ecumenical relationships with western reformation Churches. Abbot was the only Calvinist in the correspondence, but his position of influence in England was attractive to Loukaris, who became Patriarch of Constantinople in 1620. Abbot arranged for the King to support a Greek clerical student at Oxford. A monk from Mount Athos, Metrophanes Kritopoulos, came to England in 1617, and was sent by the Archbishop to Balliol. Later, Abbot disapproved of the way his theological views developed, and also disliked his need for hospitality at Lambeth, and caused him to leave the country in 1625. Communication with the Orthodox was maintained, and increased under Laud, but there was no further student in Abbot's time.[29]

Kyrillos Loukaris also corresponded with Marc' Antonio de Dominis during his stay in England. Together they hoped that King James would become the leader of all non-Roman Catholic Christians in the west, but they attributed to him more international authority than he could ever have. De Dominis had been Archbishop of Spalato[30] since 1602. He became unsettled, and after correspondence with Abbot for several years, made the journey to England in 1616, and presented himself to the King, who thriftily sent him across to Lambeth. He stayed there, studying and writing, until 1618, when he was appointed Master of the Savoy, and in the same year Dean of Windsor. On 14 December 1617, he joined Abbot and the bishops of London (J. King), Ely (L. Andrewes), Rochester (J. Buckeridge) and Lichfield (J. Overall) in the consecration at Lambeth of Nicolas Felton for Bristol and George Montaigne for Lincoln. As there were already more than the three necessary bishops present, Abbot's motives are not plain. Possibly he had the opinion of his Orthodox correspondents in mind, or perhaps it was the suggestion of the Archbishop of Spalato himself (as he continued to be called).[31] De Dominis again became unsettled, critical of Abbot's Calvinism, and disappointed that he was not given higher office, and in 1622 he returned to Italy. He was absolved by Pope Gregory XV for his separation from the Roman Church. But Gregory died in 1623. His successor, Urban VIII, was less tolerant, and de Dominis was imprisoned, and died in 1624.[32]

The Founder and His Family

An early disagreement which led to a decline in Abbot's standing in the royal favour came with the affair of the Essex divorce - or annulment. Robert Devereux, Earl of Essex, and Frances Howard, daughter of the Earl of Suffolk, were married when they were thirteen years old, in 1606. By 1609, Frances had become infatuated with Robert Carr, and in 1613 began proceedings for a decree of nullity.[33] The case was tried by a commission of which Abbot was a member. He was not convinced of the justice or honesty of the Countess's claims, and consistently opposed the termination of the marriage, despite his reluctance to take a course that conflicted with the King's wishes. To secure the desired result, James enlarged the commission. The verdict was given on 25 September, and Frances married Carr, newly created Earl of Somerset, on 26 December.[34] One immediate effect for the Abbot family was felt especially by Robert. The bishopric of Lincoln fell vacant with the death of William Barlow on 7 September. James promised the Archbishop that it should be given to Robert, but George's opposition to the King was not weakened, and his successor at Lichfield, Richard Neile, who had also been a commissioner, but in favour of the decree, was instead chosen for Lincoln.

Robert's turn for high office in the Church was not long delayed, however. On 7 May 1615 Henry Cotton, Bishop of Salisbury, died. Robert Abbot was chosen to succeed him, and was consecrated by his brother, assisted by the bishops of London (J. King), Ely (L. Andrewes) and Lincoln (R. Neile), on 3 December, the sixth anniversary of George's consecration, also in Lambeth Palace Chapel. The Archbishop spent £16.11s. on hospitality on this occasion (on wheat, beer, sack, claret, wood, coal and candles).[35] Robert resigned his Oxford professorship when he became bishop, but remained Master of Balliol until 1617.[36] He was a popular bishop, noted for his acts of charity to the poor, and to prisoners. He also raised money for repairs to the cathedral in Salisbury. Robert's wife, Maria (Deighton) died, and he displeased his brother by taking a second wife, a widow, Bridget Cheynell (Egioke). The Archbishop's opinion was governed by 2 Timothy 3,2. Robert died on 2 March 1618, aged only 58.

Archbishop Abbot did not use his patronage to advance many members of his large family of relations, but there were some who were given appointments in his service. William Kingsley, the husband of Damaris, daughter of the Archbishop's youngest brother, John, was made Archdeacon of Canterbury in 1619, and held the office for the whole of Laud's archbishopric, after Abbot's death. Nathaniel Brent, husband of Robert Abbot's daughter Martha, was helped by family influence in being elected Warden of Merton in 1622. Soon afterwards he became Vicar General to the Archbishop. He later became judge of the prerogative court of Canterbury, on the death of Sir Henry Marten, in 1641. The registrar of the court was John Abbot's son John.

Practically nothing is known about Abbot's pastoral care of his diocese of Canterbury. His predecessors had the custom of spending part of the summer in Kent, but he did not follow that policy. His first visit was in July 1615, and he went again in 1616 and 1620, and spent large sums on entertaining. In 1620 he gave a conduit to the city of Canterbury, at a cost of about £400, for the much needed improvement of the water supply. The stone pedimented and arcaded structure stood in the High Street, and was adorned with heraldry and inscriptions, and figures of the seven virtues. He intended to endow it, but a dispute with the city council caused him to change his mind.[37] After that Abbot preferred not to go further east than Croydon. For most of the time he kept good relations with the county gentry of Kent, and at the end of the law terms he invited all those who were in London to Lambeth, where he had a reputation for generous hospitality. He continued this practice until a few years before his death. There were no suffragan bishops, and confirmation cannot have been administered often. Candidates for ordination were regularly given letters dimissory, so that they might receive orders from other bishops. In 1629 and 1632 Abbot commissioned Bishop Richard Corbet to ordain on his behalf.[38] The elderly Archbishop had little time for routine diocesan duties.

Abbot found himself in another controversy in 1618. Puritan magistrates in Lancashire were attempting to force a rigid sabbatarianism onto the very mixed population. The bishop, Thomas Morton of Chester, appealed to the King for relief. James, remembering the joyless Sundays in Scotland, from which he had escaped on succeeding to the English crown, issued a declaration in 1617, permitting some social games to those who had attended church. On 24 May 1618 he extended the effect of the "Book of Sports" to the whole country, and ordered the declaration to be published in parish churches. The Archbishop was at Croydon, and forbade its reading in the church there, and this reduced still further his standing in the King's favour, to the delight of his enemies.[39]

The primate's greatest misfortune befell him in 1621. To improve his health, he took an annual holiday in Hampshire. His friend, Lord Zouche, who had congenial views on England's relations with Spain, had been rebuilding his house at Bramshill in the north of the county, and had added a chapel to the design. He invited Abbot to consecrate it, and the visit was extended into a holiday.[40] On 24 July Abbot joined a hunting party, armed with a crossbow. A keeper, Peter Hawkins, though warned of the Archbishop's probable lack of skill, ran forward. He was shot in the arm by a bolt from Abbot's bow, and quickly bled to death.

The Archbishop retired to Guildford, to await the turn of events.[41] His enemies, joined now by de Dominis, were quick to assume that the homicide, even though accidental, must disqualify him from office. King James was generous, despite their disagreement, and received Abbot back into the court in September. Nonetheless, doubt continued, and three bishops elect refused to accept consecration at his hands: John Williams, the Keeper of the Great Seal, for Lincoln, Valentine Carey for Exeter, and William Laud for St David's. To make it possible for the consecrations to take place, Abbot issued a commission to the Bishop of London, George Montaigne, who consecrated Williams on 11 November, and Carey and Laud, and also John Davenant for Salisbury, on 18 November.

On 3 October the King set up a commission of ten, consisting of lawyers and ecclesiastics, including the three bishops elect who refused to be consecrated by Abbot. Andrewes of

The Founder and His Family

Winchester was the most sympathetic to the Archbishop. The commission reported on 10 November. The members were equally divided whether the accident had made Abbot's position irregular; a majority considered that scandal might be given by it, though not intended; all agreed that the King might pardon the Archbishop and restore him to the functions of his office, though there was disagreement about the procedure. The King issued another commission to eight bishops, empowered to dispense Abbot from any irregularity, and finally a royal pardon was granted under the Great Seal, declaring that the Archbishop's position was as if the accident had never happened.

In 1622 Abbot reached his sixtieth birthday. His health was not good, and that, combined with the lack of sympathy with those in royal favour, caused him to take a less active part in the affairs of state. Nonetheless, when he considered that it was necessary, he intervened, by letter if necessary, as he did when a Spanish marriage for Prince Charles was hoped for in 1622-3. Despite the disagreements and irritations, Abbot had the respect of the King, and was called to minister to him at the end of his life.

Abbot did not lose his interest in scholarship or academic matters. When Archbishop Bancroft died in 1610, he left his books to his successors. With Sir Francis Bacon, Abbot worked out a scheme that was acceptable to the King, and Lambeth Palace Library came into being on 15 October 1612. Other libraries that benefitted by gift or bequest from George Abbot included Balliol and University Colleges at Oxford, and Canterbury and Winchester cathedrals. He gave £150 to the building of the Schools Quadrangle at Oxford, completed in 1624. His main contribution to the life of the university was in securing the foundation of Pembroke College. In 1610, Thomas Tisdale left £5000 to trustees, of whom Abbot was one, to endow additional fellows and scholars at Balliol. This was augmented by a bequest of land worth £100 annually from Richard Wightwick, for the same purpose. It was probably James I who suggested that the size of these benefactions justified the founding of a new college, incorporating Broadgates Hall, one of the most prosperous of the medieval halls, in the south-west corner of Oxford. The charter was obtained in 1624. The King was reckoned to be the founder, and the college was named after William Herbert, Earl of Pembroke, the Chancellor of the university; but it was Abbot who provided £300 to clear a debt that Balliol could not pay to the new college, so concluding the complicated negotiations.

King James died on 27 March 1625, and the consequences for Abbot of the death of Prince Henry became even more apparent, added to the hostility of the influential George Villiers, Duke of Buckingham. Williams, who was Dean of Westminster as well as Bishop of Lincoln and Keeper of the Great Seal, preached at the King's funeral on 5 May, but soon afterwards fell from favour. He resigned the Seal in October, and was not allowed to take any part in the coronation of Charles I. A commission was formed to revise the English rite prepared for James I. Abbot was a member, but the leading part was taken by Laud, who was a prebendary of Westminster as well as Bishop of St David's. The King chose Laud to take the Dean's part at the coronation on 2 February 1626, and as a bishop on the Abbey chapter, it fell to him to consecrate the chrism early in the morning.

The coronation was performed by Abbot, in poor health. Three years later, his feebleness was the reason given for Laud's action in burying Prince Charles, the first child of the King and Henrietta Maria, on 14 May 1629, the day after he was born, and baptized, and died. Laud also baptized the future Charles II a year later.

The state of the Archbishop's health prevented him from being much at court, and he spent time at Croydon, at his manor of Ford at Hoath in east Kent, and also in Guildford. His absence gave his enemies opportunity to plot against him. Two controversies about the licensing of books were used to discredit George Abbot.

The affair of Richard Montague began in about 1619, when Roman Catholics visited his parish in Essex, Stanford Rivers, and tried to convert some of the people. Montague engaged in controversy with Matthew Kellison, the president of the English College at Douay, whose book *The Gagge of the Reformed Gospell* (1623) he countered with *A Gagg for the New Gospel ? No. A New Gagg for an old Goose* (1624). His thesis was too mild for protestant opinion, as he failed to condemn Roman Catholicism unreservedly. The House of Commons denounced Montague, and requested Abbot to discipline him. The Archbishop gave him advice privately, but Montague appealed to James I, who upheld him, and arranged for a second book, *Appello Caesarem* (1625) to be licensed by Francis White, the Dean of Carlisle, without Abbot's knowledge. Abbot's protest was overtaken by the King's death. Charles I protected Montague, and appointed him a royal chaplain. After the inconclusive York House Conference at the turn of the year,[42] and the dissolution of Parliament, the matter lapsed.

The Sibthorpe affair was more serious. King Charles's relations with Parliament were sour from the beginning of his reign, and sufficient money for his needs was not voted.[43] The King sought to raise funds without the approval of Parliament, and appointed commissioners to raise forced loans. He expected the clergy to support his demand, but Abbot refused to co-operate. On 22 February 1627 Robert Sibthorpe, Vicar of St Sepulchre's Northampton, preached an assize sermon in his church, upholding the royal prerogative. The King wished the sermon to be printed, but Abbot refused to license it, on the grounds that it was not consistent with the existing law. The Archbishop persisted in his refusal, and the licence was given by the Bishop of London, George Montaigne, in May. For his defiance, Abbot was ordered in July to withdraw to his diocese. Buckingham was about to leave the country, and in order to reduce the Archbishop's already waning authority, took advantage of his bad health. He had the metropolitan jurisdiction put into commission, on 9 October, to be administered by the Bishop of London (Montaigne), Durham (Richard Neile), Bath and Wells (Laud), Oxford (John Howson) and Rochester (John Buckeridge). Despite this, Abbot continued to carry out much of his work from Croydon or Ford, through his officers. Even so, he was not allowed to preside over the consecration of Joseph Hall as Bishop of Exeter. This was done by Montaigne in his own chapel at London House on 23 December, assisted by Neile, Buckeridge and Howson, with Theophilus Field of St David's and William Murray of Kilfenora.

The Founder and His Family

Before many months had passed, the strictness of Abbot's partial suspension was allowed to relax. He attended Parliament at his fellow peers' request, but power and influence were passing to Laud, who became Bishop of London on 15 July 1628. On 24 August the Archbishop consecrated Richard Montague Bishop of Chichester in the chapel at Croydon, assisted by Laud and other bishops.[44] The ceremony was interrupted by the news of the assassination of Buckingham the day before, in Portsmouth. With his principal enemy removed, Abbot's life became easier. In December he was summoned to court, and was ceremonially conducted to the King by the Archbishop of York.[45] Charles welcomed him, and ordered him to attend the Council twice a week.

It was a sign of Laud's ascendancy that he was able, in 1629, to take the initiative in introducing reforms in the Church, of a kind that Abbot would not want. With Harsnett, the new Archbishop of York, Laud drew up regulations designed to make Church life more disciplined and orderly. They were presented by Laud to the King, who authorised them with a royal declaration, and instructed the Archbishop of Canterbury to put them into effect in the dioceses of his province. The instructions covered the residence of bishops in their dioceses and in their official houses, except when they were at court, triennial visitations by bishops, the conservation of timber in episcopal estates, the conduct of ordinations, the noting of Roman Catholics who refused to attend their parish churches, and the proper performance of public worship, including the control of church lecturers, who were often subversive of Church order and doctrine. The bishops were to make an annual report to the Archbishop.

Abbot was obliged to issue the instructions, but he did not pursue enquiries in his own diocese. When William Kingsley, Archdeacon of Canterbury and husband of Abbot's niece, attempted to act on them, the Archbishop inhibited him. On 2 January 1633 he made a report on the province to the King. He found that the Church was in good discipline, with very little to give concern. He dwelt on the Bishop of St Asaph's comments on the crowds that were flocking to St Winefrid's well at Holywell in north Wales, and reminded the King of its connexion with the gunpowder plot. He referred to one objectionable epitaph in Kent, and concluded causticly, "It may be a great comfort to your Majesty, that in so large and diffuse a Multitude both of Men and Matters, upon strict examination, there is so little exorbitancy to be found".[46]

George Abbot died in his palace at Croydon on 4 August 1633. Two days later, Laud, who had just returned from Edinburgh with Charles I, who had been crowned King of Scotland in Holyrood Palace on 18 June, received the nomination to Canterbury. It was confirmed on 19 September.

The provisions of Abbot's will, dated 25 July 1632,[47] were methodical. The poor at Lambeth and Croydon were remembered, and there were bequests to members of his family, and to friends, members of his staff, and to Princess Elizabeth, the widowed Winter Queen. Books, pictures and his barge were left to his successor, even though he knew that must be Laud.

Abbot's Hospital Guildford

The Archbishop's body was to be buried in Guildford, "that in the same town where my flesh had the beginning thereof it may rest as the *depositum* of my love to that place". The state funeral began in Croydon on 3 September, with Laud as the chief mourner and John Bowle, the Bishop of Rochester, as preacher. The body was then carried to Guildford, where it was received on 4 September by the Mayor, and taken into Holy Trinity Church for burial. In 1635 a large monument, rich in allegorical decoration, was raised over the grave by Morris Abbot. It was made by John and Matthias Christmas, probably to designs by their father Gerard , and erected by a Mr Myles.[48] In his will, George Abbot professed his confidence in "this famous Church of England which I hold to be the best framed pattern of all the Churches in Europe", and he ended beseeching "Almighty God to increase the number of the faithful, to abate more and more daily the strength of antichrist and popery; to send peace and prosperity to this island, to bless our soveraigne my most gracious lord and master the king with long life and happiness, and to send him a plentiful issue; I commend my soul again and again to the mercy of my most blessed Saviour and Redeemer".

1. The Suffolk Abbots had their relationship to the Archbishop confirmed by the College of Arms in 1664. There is information about the family in the hospital archives, probably based on the researches of J.T. Abbot FSA of Darlington, in the nineteenth century.

2. Anthony Abbot was first married in 1573, and so was probably born before the re-introduction of Latin rites in 1553-4. For details of the Guildford Abbot family, see King 1865, pp 258f.

3. This spelling, Morris, will be used for the Archbishop's brother, as it usually was in Guildford in his lifetime, to distinguish him from his father and his son.

4. D. Featley in T. Fuller: *Abel Redevivus* London 1651 p 540.

5. Story was Queen Mary's proctor at the trial of Cranmer. He was less prominent in pressing the charges than King Philip's proctor, Thomas Martin. Immediately after his execution Story was acclaimed as a Roman Catholic martyr. He was beatified on 29 December 1886 by Pope Leo XIII.

6. A. Wood: *Athenae Oxonienses* 2 ed London 1721 vol 1 col 430 (see also col 583). The cottage was an inn by 1692 and until late in the eighteenth century, the Three Mariners. It was demolished in 1864, when the wooden framed casement window was acquired by J.T. Abbot and incorporated into his house in Darlington. Mr Alan Suddes of Darlington Museum kindly identified the house, in Victoria Road, as Roseville, later called Abbeville. It was demolished in the mid-1960s, and the window was presumably destroyed. Maurice and Alice Abbot died in September 1606, and are commemorated with their sons on a brass now fixed to the south wall in Holy Trinity Church.

7. See Sturley 1980 pp 23f.

8. Matriculation at Oxford was not compulsory before 1565, when it was introduced as a means for testing loyalty to State and Church. A new Statute of Matriculation in 1581

added subscription to the Thirty-nine Articles, and in that year there was a rush of students to meet the requirements, after a period of laxity.

9. Sackville was created first Earl of Dorset on 13 March 1604. He was Lord High Treasurer from 1599 until his death.

10. For a detailed account of Abbot's publications, and their editions, see Christophers 1966.

11. The hospital has two copies, 1634 and 1636.

12. It was reprinted in 1613, and the hospital has a copy of that edition.

13. The hospital has a copy of this work, which runs to 438 pages, an example of fine Oxford printing. In 1624 most of the first section of *The Reasons* was reprinted under the title *A Treatise of the Perpetual Visibility, and Succession of the True Church in all Ages*, and issued without the author's name. The hospital has a copy.

14. The hospital has a copy of the 1611 reprint. William Perkins was a Cambridge Calvinist who published his *Reformed Catholike* in 1597, an attempt to relate Church principles to protestant theology. William Bishop was a prominent seminary priest who made several risky visits to England after his ordination in 1583. For a few months before his death in 1624 he was the first vicar apostolic for England, as Bishop of Chalcedon. His *Reformation of a Catholic Deformed by W. Perkins* began to appear in 1604.

15. The other members of the company were Richard Edes, Dean of Windsor, replaced after his death by John Aglionby, Principal of St Edmund Hall, John Harmar, Fellow of New College and Warden of Winchester College, Ralph Ravens, Fellow of St John's, later replaced by Leonard Hutton, Canon of Christchurch, Thomas Ravis, Dean of Christchurch until 1605, then Bishop of Gloucester until 1607 and of London until his death in 1609, Henry Savile, the only layman, Warden of Merton and Provost of Eton, and Giles Thomson, Fellow of All Souls and Dean of Windsor.

16. 26 May. It was published, and there is a copy at the hospital.

17. For a summary account of Bancroft's policies, see Carpenter 1971 pp 176-8.

18. This was recorded by Peter Heylin, an admirer of Laud and not of Abbot, and may not be a fair report. *Cyprianus Anglicus* London 1668 p 244.

19. Samuel Harsnett, later Archbishop of York, was consecrated Bishop of Chichester at the same time.

20. This Abbot succession in Scotland did not endure. In 1638 the General Assembly voted to abolish episcopacy, and all the bishops were deprived on 13 December. Only one lived until the Restoration, Thomas Sydserf of Galloway, but he took no part in later consecrations. He did, however, ordain many men to the priesthood after the restoration, to the annoyance of the English bishops, so that they could be qualified to hold benefices. The episcopate in Scotland was restored again in 1661, when Bishop Gilbert Sheldon of London consecrated four bishops, from whom the succession has continued.

21. The last previous Archbishop of Canterbury to serve longer than that was William Warham, 1503-1532; and the next was Charles Manners-Sutton, 1805-1828.

22. E. Hyde: *The History of the Rebellion and Civil Wars begun in the Year 1641* Oxford 1702 vol 1 p 68.

23. Welsby 1962 has useful comments on the High Commission pp 43-6.

24. Davies 1959 gives a useful discussion pp 205-10. Early in his reign, James even hoped that the Pope, Clement VIII, would summon an ecumenical council, and invite representatives of the Church of England and of the north European protestant churches. See Patterson 1971 pp 267-275 for James's moves in this area of church relations.

25. The Roman Catholic martyrs - 1610: Roger Cadwallador, George Napper, John Roberts, Thomas Somers; 1612: William Scott, Richard Newport, St John Almond; 1614: John Mawson; 1616: Thomas Atkinson, John Thules, Roger Wrenno, Thomas Maxfield, Thomas Tunstall; 1618: William Southerne; 1628 St Edmund Arrowsmith, Richard Hurst. For biographical notes and aliases see Walsh and Barry 1979, and Foley 1987.

26. The Lord Treasurer, Robert Cecil, arranged to have Sir George More of Loseley, Guildford, appointed treasurer to the Prince in an effort to curb his expenditure, but he did not succeed.

27. A.P. Stanley: *Historical Memorials of Westminster Abbey* London 1868 p 175.

28. Welsby 1962 gives an account of these negotiations pp 51f, 80, 83f, 107-13.

29. For Loukaris see Strenopoulos 1951. The Patriarch was murdered in 1638. For Kritopoulos see Davey 1987.

30. Now Split, in Yugoslavia. From the foundation of the bishopric in 653 the mausoleum of the Emperor Diocletian (died 316) has been used as the cathedral.

31. As Montaigne presided over the consecration of Laud, assisted by Felton, the part de Dominis took on 14 December 1617 has had significance for the nature of the episcopal succession in the Church of England.

32. For de Dominis see Malcolm 1984. Malcolm states, p 64, that de Dominis stressed the importance of the apostolic succession, which he believed the Church of England had retained. Malcolm does not, however, mention the consecration of Felton and Montaigne.

33. The case is well described in Welsby 1962 pp 57-73.

34. During Lent 1631, before the death of Frances, Essex married Elizabeth Paulet. The shortlived son of the marriage was born and baptized at Loseley in 1636, and registered in the same book at Guildford St Nicolas as the baptism of George Abbott.

35. This may be compared with £4.13.6d for George Carleton, consecrated for Llandaff in 1618, and £1.18.4d for Robert's second successor, Robert Townson, in 1620 (both in the summer, when wood, coal and candles could be spared, which had cost £1.19.10d in December 1615 for Robert); also with the 2d that the Archbishop regularly sent to the church outside his palace gate for the Sunday collection.

36. He was succeeded at Balliol by John Parkhurst, of a Guildford family. Residence in Oxford would have been convenient for visiting the northern part of the diocese of Salisbury, which at that time included Berkshire.

The Founder and His Family

37. The wooden water pipes quickly decayed, and the conduit fell into disrepair. In 1754 it was decided that it obstructed traffic and it was demolished. The water tank was resited above St George's gateway, which, in turn, was pulled down in 1800-1.

38. Corbet, Bishop of Oxford 1628~32, and of Norwich 1632-5, came from Ewell, Surrey.

39. Charles I reissued the "Book of Sports" on 18 October 1633, after Abbot's death in August.

40. Bramshill House is now the Police Staff College, and what remains of Lord Zouche's chapel was rededicated for Roman Catholic use by Cardinal Heenan on 19 March 1964.

41. Abbot sorrowed for this accident for the rest of his life, and fasted once a month in reparation. He made an annual allowance of £20 to the widow of Hawkins, and left her an annuity of this amount in his will. With this endowment she was able to find another husband.

42. For a brief comment on the York House Conference see Collinson 1982 p 34.

43. For the relations between Charles I and his early parliaments, see Davies 1959 pp 34-46.

44. The consecration of Joseph Hall for Exeter in 1627 was the only one performed by the commission. Abbot resumed this office with the consecration of Montague, and presided over all consecrations for the province of Canterbury, except that of John Owen for St Asaph in 1629, until the end of his life.

45. Samuel Harsnett, nominated as Archbishop, but not confirmed until 13 January 1629. He had been consecrated with Abbot in 1609.

46. The instructions, and Abbot's account of the province for 1632, are printed in *The History of the Troubles and Tryal of the Most Reverend Father in God and Blessed Martyr, William Laud* London 1695 pp 517-20.

47. The will is printed in A.Onslow: *The Life of Dr. George Abbot*, (reprinted with some additions and corrections from the *Biographia Britannica*) Guildford 1777 pp 57-72, from which the quotations are taken.

48. P.G. Palmer, in *The Knight of the Red Cross* Guildford 1911, explains the mystery of the tomb, considering it to be based on Edmund Spenser's *Faerie Queene*. The tomb stood in the north-east corner of the ancient church, over the grave, which is therefore at the north-east corner of the present nave. The monument survived the collapse of the tower and much of the church in 1740. It was moved eastwards into the new south transept, built in 1888. During this building work, the vault was accidentally opened, and "the form of the body clearly revealed, and the beard still apparently intact". (Williamson 1904 has a description of this event p 115.) As early as 1646 the tomb was hung round with "Greene Bayse" curtains - fifteen yards of material provided by the hospital for 35/-d. Later black curtains were favoured.

Abbot's Hospital Guildford

TWO
THE FOUNDATION

The word "hospital" as we use it in the name of our institution, carries a meaning nearer to its origin than when it denotes a place for the care of the sick. Hospitality is a Christian duty, enjoined by Christ (St Matthew 25,35), and encouraged by the leaders of the Church. In the fifth century it was realised that gifts to poor travellers were not enough, and that sometimes shelter was needed. In the fourth century, after the peace of the Church, the *xenodochia* had become known, a hostel for strangers, later called *hospitium* or *hospitale*. Imperial and Church authority encouraged these foundations, and bishops were urged to see that there were enough of them. As they became more formally established they housed those who needed to stay longer, or permanently, and so the care of the sick was also undertaken.[1]

In England hospitals were found before the Norman conquest. The names of five are known, the earliest being St Peter's York, founded by King Athelstan in about 937. Only one of the preconquest hospitals survives, St Oswald's Worcester, founded before 972, now in buildings of 1873-4.[2] During the medieval period there were about a thousand hospital foundations in England. Some were short-lived, and either failed, or were combined with others. In the fourteenth century, before the Black Death, there were nearly seven hundred open, but then came a decline, and by the fourth decade of the sixteenth century the number had fallen probably to less than five hundred.[3] Although their main purpose was to give shelter and care to those who stayed there, and in some cases medical attention, they were religious houses, and those who supervised them often lived under rule, usually a form of the rule of St Augustine. As permanent residence began to be provided, and the almshouse style of hospital developed, those who lived there formed a sort of community, and statutes laid down directions for their common life and worship. The most famous of all the medieval hospitals is St Cross at Winchester, founded before 1137. An early example of the courtyard plan is the almshouse at Ewelme, in Oxfordshire, founded in 1437.

Many hospitals were connected with chantries - endowed masses for the dead, and this was sufficient reason for their suppression under Edward VI, many already having fallen to Henry VIII. But care for the sick and the aged poor was still needed, and efforts were made to rescue the hospitals, and secure their future. Some were able to carry on without much change, others were altered, or refounded after an interval, with their purposes more precisely defined. St Bartholomew's at Smithfield, for example, was changed without a break in 1544 from a religious institution for the sick and for travellers into a secular hospital for the sick. One of those which escaped dissolution was a small hospital in Guildford, which Abbot knew from childhood.

Abbot's Hospital Guildford

St Thomas's Hospital was in existence before 1214. It was founded as an asylum for those who suffered from leprosy, but as the disease became less common it changed into a home for the poor. It stood, as a leprosy hospital would, outside the town boundary, in the angle of the junction of the London and Epsom roads. Dedications to St Thomas Becket were not approved at the time of the reformation, and the little house became known as the Spital, and gave its name to the road approaching it from the town. By the seventeenth century the charity supported only one resident, known as the prior, and it came to an end in the eighteenth century.[4] When Abbot was considering how to use some of his bachelor wealth[5] for a permanent charity, he knew that Croydon was well provided for, and he was not likely to do more for Canterbury. Lambeth does not seem to have been considered, and he turned to his native town. He knew that there was no need to provide a school, as he had been well educated there himself at the Free Grammar School, and there was also Thomas Baker's School. He could have re-established the Spital, but he decided to undertake a more ambitious scheme, of which a hospital was only a part.

The Archbishop was able to learn from the close connexions he had with several foundations, and wrote in chapter 11 of the Guildford statutes "experience in other places hath taught me..." Robert Sackville, Earl of Dorset, son of Abbot's patron Thomas, the first Earl, died in 1609, leaving money to build a hospital with an endowment at East Grinstead. Abbot was a member of the commission that finally succeeded in building Sackville College and securing the approval of the statutes. Thomas Sutton, founder of the Hospital of King James in the London Charterhouse - a hospital and school, died in 1611. Abbot was one of the overseers of his will, and chairman of the body which compiled the statutes. Abbot knew about about Edward Alleyn's College of God's Gift at Dulwich, a school and almshouse, and had dedicated the chapel in 1616, during the vacancy of the see of Winchester. Perhaps he knew Richard Wyatt of Shackleford, who died in 1619, leaving a bequest that built Wyatt's Almshouses at Godalming. But it was at Croydon that he was able to learn most, from the Whitgift Foundation.

John Whitgift (c 1530-1604) was Archbishop of Canterbury from 1583 until his death. As a child he gained the interest of his uncle, Robert Whitgift, the last Abbot of Wellow, a small but orderly Augustinian house near Grimsby, dissolved in 1536. Whitgift therefore grew up knowing something of the traditions of the life of a religious community, and this influence was seen in the statutes of his foundation. He decided that Croydon, where he often stayed in his manor house (first called a palace in his time) should be the place where he set up his charity, though it was also to serve Lambeth. He received the royal licence in November 1595. Two months later the building began, and Whitgift laid the foundation stone on 22 March 1596. The chapel was dedicated on 9 July 1599 by Bishop Bancroft of London, and the hospital was finished that September. The school, which opened in 1600, was nearby.

The hospital consists of one quadrangle, with rooms originally for thirty-two brothers and sisters. The main rooms are on the opposite side of the courtyard to the principal entrance. The chapel is in the right hand corner, and the common hall is to the left. Above it is the audience chamber and other rooms for the Archbishop's own use, in which he was succeeded by the wardens. In this foundation the most important official was the schoolmaster, who also acted as chaplain. The warden was elected by the brothers from among themselves. Abbot, who also lived frequently at Croydon, knew the hospital and school well. In 1616 he held a visitation, through commissioners, and expelled the schoolmaster, and one of the brothers.

Abbot became Archbishop in 1611. Three years later he had begun to think what charitable foundation he should make. He thought then that he would not be able to afford anything on the scale of the Whitgift Foundation, so he decided that he should attempt to support the cloth industry, the main trade of Guildford and of his own family. Through Tudor times the manufacture and sale of English woollen cloth had expanded, but early in the seventeenth century there was a recession. Trade was adversely affected by wars in northern Europe; new textiles were reducing the demand for wool; and production in small towns was overtaken by London business practices.[6] On 14 December 1614 Abbot wrote to the Mayor of Guildford with his proposal. The poor would be more easily looked after if the town were more prosperous. He had heard of a scheme practised in the Low Countries, where grants were made to poor workmen to help them build or improve their looms. He would make an endowment, which would produce income to provide not grants but loans, free of interest, to help poor clothworkers improve their businesses. With the letter he sent £100, but it was not to be used until he came to Guildford. Loans were made from this sum at least until 1623, but by then Abbot had discovered that he could be considerably more generous than he had thought.

By 1618 the Archbishop had made his plans, and began to make preparations for a double foundation, a hospital and a "manufacture". He acquired the site, running from the High Street to what is now North Street. The Half Moon inn was bought from Robert Purse for £350 in April 1618. Property to the east of the inn was bought from Henry Astrete for £100 in the following October.[7] The land and the buildings, which were to be demolished, were purchased in the name of trustees, Sir Nicholas Kempe of Islington,[8] William Baker of Lambeth, the Archbishop's secretary, and Morris Abbot his brother. The site is not rectangular, and this caused a pleasant irregularity to the plan of the buildings.

In April 1618 George Austen, former mayor and member of Parliament for Guildford,[9] was commissioned by Abbot to spend £100 in buying timber for the hospital. Apart from that practically nothing is known about the building work. The first stone was laid on 6 April 1619 by the Archbishop,[10] who was accompanied by his friend Sir Nicholas Kempe. Abbot regarded Kempe as the principal benefactor of the hospital, and the money spent on timber was his gift. When he died, in 1624, he left to Abbot plate to the value of £500, and this was devoted to the purchase of land for the endowment. The building was sufficiently advanced for Abbot to stay there for a while after the death of Peter Hawkins in July 1621, and ready for full use by October 1622. 1621 is marked in black flints at the north end of the garden wall. Building continued until 1631, when the turrets were completed.[11] Some of the rainwater-heads are dated 1627.

Following Whitgift's example, the Guildford hospital was planned round a courtyard, entered through a gatehouse tower, in which, as at Croydon, there was a secure room for the records of the foundation. At Guildford there was the additional safeguard that the "evidence house" could be entered only by way of the master's lodging. The chapel was placed in the far right hand corner, rising the height of two storeys, as Whitgift's chapel did, but here the axis is in line with the far range of the quadrangle, so that the altar is at the east end. The common hall is west of the chapel. To the west of the hall a passage goes through the building, and on its left is a staircase leading to the guesten hall. At the end of the passage the falling land makes a flight of steps necessary to reach the large garden, which was intended to produce food for the hospital. The master's lodgings were placed in the eastern end of the front range, with the main room over the gateway. Abbot gave himself the right to occupy these rooms whenever he wished to stay in Guildford, and then the master was to move across to the north-west corner.[12] The rooms for the eight women were on the left, or west side of the courtyard, and the twelve brothers' rooms were on the right.

The quality of Abbot's building is very high. The hospital is planned on a grand scale, and the detail is fine, especially the woodwork. Abbot's presence chamber over the gateway, now the Governors' boardroom, is panelled to the ceiling, and is a very impressive appartment, as it was intended to be.

The chapel windows appear to shew a change in design. What remained of the Dominican friary in Guildford was demolished early in the seventeenth century by Sir George More of Loseley, a friend of Abbot, and it would be true to the Archbishop's character while building an expensive structure, to beg or bargain for two spare windows, when he had decided to introduce stained glass. The glass was probably designed and partly made by Baptista Sutton, and the date 1621 appears at the top of the north window. The main lights contain scenes from the life of the patriarch Jacob (perhaps as a compliment to James I), beginning in the four-light north window, and continuing in the five-light east window. The headlights contain heraldic displays, in the east window referring to the royal family, and in the north window shewing the episcopal career of George Abbot.[13]

It is not clear when the new hospital buildings were put into use. As has been stated, Abbot himself stayed there in the late summer of 1621. In April 1622 a letter was addressed to the "Master and brethren of the Hospitall of the Blessed Trinity in Guilford", although the corporate body had not been set up. It may be that the Archbishop had installed his eldest brother, Richard, as a caretaker, and allowed some of the rooms to be occupied. In 1622, Abbot decided that his sixtieth birthday should be the official time for the new foundation to be inaugurated. Letters patent were obtained from James I on 20 June, and on 29 October, the controller of the Archbishop's household, Richard Brigham, arrived from Lambeth. He called together the Mayor, Richard Burchall, the

The Foundation

previous Mayor, Robert Terry, the Rector of Holy Trinity, John Wright, and several other townsmen. After prayers in the chapel, the letters patent were displayed, and received as the hospital's royal charter.[14] Richard Abbot was declared the first Master. He took the oath of royal supremacy, and the oath of the master, and the charter was given into his keeping. Richard was then seventy-three years old, and had been a widower for over twelve years.

On the same day that the first master was installed, five brothers were admitted to the hospital, George Burges, Gregory Frye, Richard Butcher, Robert George Kitchiner and John Rapley. A sixth, Richard Pardye had been a servant of the founder's parents, as had his first wife. However, he had married again, and so was not eligible for admission. He was given a brother's allowance, and it was decided that when he or his wife died, the survivor should be admitted. Pardye was the first to benefit from Abbot's intention that founder's kin, and those who had served his father or himself, should be capable of admission to the hospital, even if they did not qualify by age or residence in Guildford. Pardye's room was given to James Seaman, who was the first brother to die, on 26 March 1623. The first sisters were admitted on 14 March 1623, Joan Rapley, Emlin Martin, Winifred Harte and Jane Heath, all widows. Further admissions followed, to increase the number, or to replace residents who had died or left, and by the end of May 1626 the hospital was full. Of the first brothers, George Burges lived until December 1632, and of the first five sisters, Winifred Harte until July 1635.

The hospital, with the land on which it was built, was conveyed from the trustees to the Master and Brethren on 26 June 1624, for the price of five shillings. For the first few years the hospital had no statutes, and it was not adequately endowed. The Archbishop kept a close watch on its affairs, and to start with had to pay for most of the expenses. He intended that the life of the community should be similar to that of Whitgift's Hospital at Croydon, and it may be that the Croydon statutes were used at first in Guildford. Some variations were found to be necessary, and some points were dictated by his own habits and interests, such as the banning of dogs, "for the better preserving of all the glasse in the Howse". By 1629 Abbot was ready to give the statutes to his foundation, and he signed them on 17 August, in the presence of Sir Morris Abbot his brother, Sir Morris's son Maurice, Richard Brigham and Walter Dobson.[15]

The hospital was founded for the benefit of single people in need, who had been born in the town of Guildford, or who had lived there for twenty years. Abbot was questioned about the area of benefit, and it was suggested that he should include the rural part of the very large parish of St Nicolas. He was emphatic in insisting that he meant the town as it was in 1620 – "under the governement of the Maior, and my desire was and is, to keepe my Charitie within boundes". *"May I not do what I will with mine owne?"*[16]

Those who were admitted as brothers and sisters were to be not less than sixty years of age, of good health and character, and preference was to be given to those who had served the town as office-bearers or in business, or who had fought for their country. Abbot reserved the selection of residents to himself, and it may be imagined that he acted on the advice of friends or members of his family living in Guildford. After the founder's death, choice of new brothers and sisters was to be made, within a day of vacancies occurring, by the Mayor or his deputy, and by the master alternately. If the master was absent, his turn was taken by the master of the Grammar School. If the choice was not made within twenty-four hours, the Mayor's nomination lapsed to the Rector of St Nicolas', and the master's to the Rector of Holy Trinity - unless the Rector was himself the master, in which case it would lapse to the Rector of St Mary's. Each nomination was to be announced in the chapel, in the presence of at least four residents, and then the new member was led to the room that was vacant. For three months the newcomer did not receive any allowance. At the end of that time the oaths were to be taken, and then the brother or sister was qualified to have a share in the distribution of money. The room in the south-west corner of the courtyard, larger than the rest, was to be occupied by a person who had held some office in the town.

It might happen that there was no single man or woman in the town suitable and eligible for a vacant place in the hospital. In that case a married man or woman might be chosen, with the approval of the Mayor and the Rector of Holy Trinity, to be an out-brother or out-sister. Such a member of the hospital would receive the allowances, but have no right to occupy a room.

The special provision for relations of Abbot, and for those who had been servants of the Archbishop or his father, was taken up several times. The statutes limited them to three of each category at any time. When Abbot nominated a brother or sister he was not bound by his own rules, and men younger than sixty were admitted from time to time. A note in the ledger against the admission of Caleb Keyes in 1626 hints at disapproval of this indulgence. "Nonethelesse it was his Graces owne pleasure in this case & for this pson to dispense wth the statute of the house, Not intending That his admission beinge wthin age shalbe a president hereafter." With him was admitted John Tegge, who seems to have left immediately. Tegge was admitted again, and was then only forty years of age. He proved a trouble-maker. Within the period of his probation he received his first admonition in the chapel, for drunkenness and brawling. Three years later he received his second admonition, for attempting to hang himself, or pretending to. When he was cut down he threatened to do it again, but he died early in 1635.

The Archbishop hoped that the hospital would be a quiet and peaceful place - but he knew that there must be a system of discipline, with penalties for those who disturbed the lives of their fellows. His rules were based on those laid down by Whitgift for the Croydon hospital. Any found guilty of a criminal offence must be expelled. Offences causing scandal or disorder in the hospital were to be dealt with by admonitions, which were to be recorded in the ledger. The first was a warning. The second was strengthened by the forfeit for a month of all financial benefit. The third brought expulsion. Admonitions were regularly recorded for such things as brawling, swearing, fighting, drunkenness, and disrespectful language to the master.

The Foundation

Abbot declared himself the Visitor of the hospital, and he was to be followed by his successors as Archbishop of Canterbury. Abbot was also to appoint the master, but after his death, an election was to be held when the mastership fell vacant. The five electors were the Mayor or his deputy, the Rector of Holy Trinity, or, in his absence, the Rector of St Nicolas', the vice-master and the two senior brethren. The election was to be held within twenty-four hours of the vacancy's being known. If it was not completed in that time, it lapsed to the Archbishop for twelve days, then to the Bishop of Winchester for seven days, then to Sir George More of Loseley or his successor in that estate, for five days. If still no appointment was made, the choice returned to the electors. The master must have been born in Guildford, or have lived there for twenty years, and be over fifty years of age, and single. If a master married, he was to leave within three days. Single men who had served as Mayor were eligible for election, and so was the Rector of Holy Trinity, if unmarried, even if he had not been born in Guildford. If a master was found to be negligent, a report was to be made to the Archbishop of Canterbury, who would decide what action to take. The yearly payment of the master was to be £20.

A vice-master was to be appointed on the last day of September every year, chosen by the master and the five senior brethren in residence. His payment for the year was thirteen shillings and fourpence. The office of porter was held in turn for a month by the five junior brothers. The porter locked and unlocked the gate, and rang the bell for prayers. The sisters were to share the duty of caring for the sick, but two were to be appointed every year on 30 September, to have special responsibility as "Releevers of the impotent", and each was paid six shillings and eightpence for the year. If a woman refused this task, she was to forfeit all financial emoluments in the hospital for the whole year. This severe rule was one of the passages copied from Whitgift's statutes. Office-bearers and some senior brothers had the responsibility of keeping the keys. In particular the evidence house over the entrance, and the chests in which money and documents were to be kept, could only be approached when several people were present with their keys. As was the case at the Croydon hospital, the statutes did not provide for a cook. The brothers and sisters were responsible for their own meals, and no doubt saw that the sick and incapable did not go hungry.

Abbot was intent upon founding a community, not simply a group of residences. The chapel was to have central importance, and prayers were to be read there daily, morning and evening. On Sundays, festivals, Wednesdays and Fridays, all the residents were to walk in twos across the road, morning and evening (and on Saturday evenings as well) to Holy Trinity Church to worship there, and to receive Holy Communion at least three times a year. Persistent absentees were to be punished with fines, or ultimately with expulsion. Whitgift's hospital had similar rules, but Abbot added the comment, "Whie should any one who will not serve God, be thought fitt to be in this Body". The chapel was also used for the election of the master, for announcing the nomination of brothers and sisters, and for the annual reading of the statutes on the Wednesday in Easter week.[17]

Abbot's Hospital Guildford

The social life of the hospital was to be strengthened by four feasts every year, at Christmas, Easter, Whitsun, and on the founder's birthday. A sense of community was also to be reinforced by the wearing of gowns. These were to be made every other autumn, "a large Gowne" for the master, and "a reasonable gowne according to the tallnesse or stature of the partie that is to weare it" for each brother and sister. The first gowns were not bought with hospital funds, but were provided in 1626 from the legacy of Edward Ayleworth, of Hackington in Kent. Abbot intended that the master and residents should regard the hospital as their home, and regularly be there, without "much flitting abroade". He allowed two months' absence in a year, but no-one should lodge in Guildford, away from the hospital. These rules for residence were similar to those at Whitgift's hospital.

The Archbishop encouraged brothers and sisters to seek employment of a suitable kind. The keeping of "any Ale-house or Vicualing howse" was specified as unsuitable, and forbidden. Crafts might be pursued in the hospital itself, so long as no annoyance was caused to the other residents. Begging was strictly forbidden. Brothers and sisters who broke windows, or caused other damage, were to repair them at their own expense. Unaccountable damage in the public rooms was to be put right at the hospital's charge. Every year, on the Monday following the festival of the Nativity of St John Baptist (24 June) the master was to choose three brothers, and make a thorough inspection of the whole of the building and its grounds, and set in hand any necessary repairs. Urgent matters, such as dislodged tiles, should be seen to straight away, whatever the time of year. Characteristically, Abbot ordered that every Saturday afternoon, the chapel and hall must be swept by the three junior sisters in turn, who should also bring in herbs and flowers from the garden, when they were available, to decorate them. He added that no "swine or other noisome beast" must be kept in the hospital garden, "because my desire is that both comelinesse and health should bee every way preserved". Furthermore, "for the better preserving of all the glasse in the Howse, I do vtterly forbid the keeping of any Dogge within the Hospitall or precincts thereof, vpon paine, (to the partie offending) of forfeiting Five shillings to the Common Chest for every daye. And in this I require the Maister and Vice-maister vpon their oath to be very severe."

The endowment of the hospital was to be secured by rents from land which Abbot bought. The first purchase was in 1622, the year that the first master and brothers were admitted. On 10 April John Harwood wrote to the master and brethren saying that he had heard from Sir George More of Loseley that the Archbishop had heard that Harwood's farm at Merrow was for sale, and that he was offering £1700 for it. Hall Place farm and a number of detached fields at Merrow and elsewhere comprised two hundred and fifteen acres, and produced a yearly income of £100. Harwood said that the farm was worth £2000, in "iust and answerable dealing a pennyworth for a penny". The sale price was agreed at £1800. In 1625 Rumbeams at Ewhurst was bought, about ninety acres for £550, from Thomas Hill. Early in 1626 Mereden at Dorking was bought, about three hundred acres for £1040, from Edward Goodwyn. Later in 1626, Highlands at Horsham was purchased, one hundred and seventy acres for £400, from the Constable family. The

The Foundation

rents from these four properties were to bring in £187.10s (Merrow £80, Rumbeams £27.10s, Mereden £40, Highlands £40), only a little short of the £200 that Abbot considered sufficient income.[18] The remaining £12.10s was to pay for fuel. Some land, the Woodlands at St Catherine's in the parish of St Nicolas, was bought in 1629, and should have provided the fuel money. It was found to be an unreliable source of income, and Abbot soon looked for another arrangement. In 1631 he considered buying Brooklands in Chiddingfold, thirty acres for £140. He changed his mind, and bought the manor of West Wantley, at Stillington in Sussex, in 1632. Its income was a rent of £44.10s, and after providing the charge for fuel in the hospital, left £32 for the Archbishop. These details were not settled by the time of Abbot's death, and there was a dispute, which will be mentioned in a later chapter.[19] The rents of all the farms were paid regularly until 1630, when James Harwood was found to owe £10 for Merrow, and he continued in arrears. The farms were made over to the Master and Brethren by a deed of endowment on 11 July 1629.

The largest part of the income, £130, was for the weekly distribution of two shillings and sixpence to each brother and sister. The payment of the master and other office-holders amounted to £22.6.8d, and the Rector of Holy Trinity was to receive thirty shillings. The four gaudy days were endowed with ten shillings each. About £15 was to be set aside each year for making gowns for the master and residents. New ones were to be made every two years. If a brother or sister died, the gown was to be given to the successor to the vacancy. When necessary some money might be spent on fuel, to supplement the £12.10s secured for that purpose. Abbot thriftily reminded the master that when buying "sea-cole, or Charcole", he should do it "in the Somer time, it will be the cheaper, because the wayes are fairer". He hoped that another economy could be achieved by cutting wood at St Catherine's, which was in possession when the statutes were given. The balance of the revenue, which might be increased by fines, and by the accumulation of the weekly distribution when not all the places were filled, was to be kept "for the stock of the House", available for repairs, legal expenses and other outgoings. When a reserve of £100 was reached, it was to be converted into gold. Its existence was to be kept secret.

Like Whitgift,[20] Abbot made detailed regulations for the paying of rents, and for the regulation of leases, which were not to be longer than twenty-one years. The responsibilities of tenants were clearly defined. When leases were renewed, the fines were to be divided. Half was to be put into the treasury; the other half was to be shared among the master and residents, with a double portion for the master. Abbot ordered that the rents of the farms were not to be increased, except that if one fell in value, the balance could be kept by adding to the others. In assuming a permanently stable economy he was misled, and this caused difficulties for his foundation in the years that followed.

The annual account was to be made on 29 October, the Archbishop's birthday, and to be completed by 1 November. (The financial year ran from 29 September, Michaelmas.) The statement was to be declared to the community, for the praise or blame of those who managed the hospital's affairs, according to whether surplus or deficit was found. The Archbishop wrote, a little smugly, "There is nothing that maketh any *Corporation* so to florish, as good husbandry, and diligent looking to the state thereof; And if I your Founder in the course of my life had not been provident in that way, how should I have been able to builde this House, and endow it with possessions."

Not much is known about the first master, Richard Abbot. He married Eden Banister at Holy Trinity on 3 May 1573. Six children were baptized at Holy Trinity, five sons, two of whom died in infancy, and a daughter. Eden Abbot died in May 1610. Richard Abbot kept no records of the management of the hospital until the end of his mastership. He was an old man, and his brother very probably appointed him as an act of kindness and respect to the head of his family. On 8 November 1623, the hospital chapel was used for the baptism of the master's grandson, Thomas Abbot.[21]

Richard Brigham came to Guildford on 21 August 1629. It is certain that he brought with him the newly sealed deed of endowment and book of statutes, and that he explained how the funds were to be managed. He checked the accounts and left £38.12s for the regular expenses of the quarter, and told Richard to pay future bills from the endowment income. Nonetheless, when money was required to pay for two feather beds and bolsters (13.6d) and a chest with drawer boxes (£4.15s), the master sent to Lambeth for it as he always had. Perhaps he thought that these were extraordinary expenses, but Brigham wrote again on 6 November 1629, repeating the instruction that the hospital must pay its way. This letter also spoke of the Archbishop's displeasure at hearing that the master was using rooms in the hospital for storing corn – an abuse that must stop. Richard Abbot saw that he must conduct affairs according to the statutes, and arranged for John Champion to start the first statement of account. Champion opened a clean page some way into the ledger, and began "Thaccompt of Mr Richard Abbatt Warden then taken the 13th November Anno Dni 1629". Under "charge" he entered the rents that Brigham had left, £38.12s, and £7 due from Sir George More, fuel money from St Catherine's. Under "discharge" were the allowances for the residents, payments to the "warden", vice-master, the Rector of Holy Trinity, the sisters who cared for the sick, and the clerk. Ten shillings was paid for the dinner on 29 October, and sixpence quitrent for the forecourt, to the bailiff. The payment for fuel was outstanding, as the money had not been received. The expenses exceeded the income by twopence, which was struck off in the ledger – and there was no mention of the chest or the bedding. The master had to learn to carry accounts from one quarter to another, as money became available.

Before the next account Richard Abbot had died, on 2 March 1630. He was buried at Holy Trinity two days later. The Archbishop wrote to the Mayor of Guildford on 24 March, thanking him for the care taken over the master's funeral. He promised that Richard's successor should be more capable of managing the business of the hospital – "a fitt Governour ... a man of some learninge & good experience who may by his paynes establish that wch my Brother by reason of his educacon otherwise was not hable to pforme".

The Foundation

As the second master, Abbot chose Jasper Yardley, whom he knew well. Yardley had been for several years in Archbishop Bancroft's service at Lambeth, and later, from 13 December 1621, warden of the hospital at Croydon, which he resigned on 19 March 1630, still aged only fifty. In his letter of appointment (the same in which he mentioned the first master's funeral) the Archbishop added a simple ceremony to the manner of receiving a new master in the chapel laid down in the statutes. Before taking the oaths, he was to read the statute concerning the master. After the oaths, the Mayor or his deputy was "to bringe him to the Lodginge, whc my Brother had, & putting him therin to Leave him in the same". This was done on 25 March 1630, recorded in the ledger by John Champion, and attested by the Mayor, Robert Terry, and by Thomas Parkhurst and John Crane.

On the day of his admission, Yardley began to take careful control of the hospitals affairs, leaving a record in the ledger, which he kept in his own hand, more neatly than Champion had. Admissions were recorded in the front, with the accumulation of "dead pay" noted in each case. He continued the accounts after Champion's entry, and used the same method. On the left hand page he recorded all the money received and due to the hospital on the day of his admission. On the right hand page he entered expenditure for the following period. Because it was six months until the first Michaelmas account he fell into the habit of making the reckoning every half year, instead of annually as the statutes required. Near to the back of the book Yardley entered the admonitions of brothers and sisters. He began by recording the earlier admonition of Caleb Keyes in Richard Abbot's mastership, shewing that he had noted him as a trouble-maker.

Ordinary repairs are noted, of the sort that have continued ever since, and maintenance expenses, as when two men were paid one shilling and eightpence for three quarters of a day's work, clearing the roof and gutters. The turrets were not complete, and Yardley was evidently not satisfied with the way that they were covered, for he borrowed one hundred and fifty slates from the Mayor, and spent three halfpence for nails for fixing them up. In 1631 the slates were returned to the Mayor, and the lead ogee roofs were set up on the turrets. So Yardley finished the building of the hospital, within the lifetime of the founder.[22] On his own part, George Abbot renewed his intentions for the hospital and manufacture in his will, stating that if there was any defect in the conveying of any of the farms for the endowment, they were to be given by his executors, as a bequest.

1. For the early development of hospitals see Nasalli-Rocca 1967 pp 159-63, and Ullmann 1971 pp 9-12.
2. The others are St Mary and St Andrew Flixton, North Yorkshire (before 940), Holy Trinity Stow-on-the-Wold, Gloucestershire (c 1010) and St Nicholas Pontefract, West Yorkshire (before 1066). St Peter's York was later called St Leonard's.
3. For lists of the hospitals and other details see Knowles and Hadcock 1971.

Abbot's Hospital Guildford

4. Some time after 1628 the Spital became part of the Poyle Trust. When it ceased to be a hospital, the site was used to produce an income for the trust. It was eventually sold, in 1932, for £11,000. Drawings of the hospital as it was in 1791 are reproduced in Williamson 1904. The accompanying text is more inaccurate even than most of the rest of this book.

5. There was no archbishop's wife at Lambeth from the death of Mrs Parker in 1570 until the arrival of Mrs Tillotson in 1691. With no children to provide for, the primates could be generous in provision for the poor, and for the pursuit of learning.

6. The state of the cloth trade is discussed in Davies 1959 pp 288-93.

7. £450 was a large sum, but a prime site in Guildford was not to be had cheaply even in the early seventeenth century.

8. Kempe was steward of the episcopal manors of Fulham, and was knighted by James I in 1617.

9. George Austen was the sort of man to win Abbot's trust and admiration - successful, and a benefactor of the Grammar School. See Sturley 1980 passim.

10. The stone, with very crudely cut lettering, is now in the chapel wall, hidden by the altar, put there in 1931.

11. The turrets had been left unfinished because they were inclining inwards as the tower shrank. Time was allowed for the brickwork to settle.

12 Abbot was less demanding than Whitgift, who retained three rooms for his own use. After his death they were to be kept for his executors for one year, and then for his brother George Whitgift. Only after that did they become the warden's lodging.

13. The glass is discussed in Rackham 1947-51 pp 5-8.

14. The charter hangs framed, with its seal, in the boardroom. The common seal of the hospital was made in 1622, ready for use for the business of the endowments.

15. The sealed book of the statutes is still kept in the strongroom of the hospital. An edition was published by P.G. Palmer in 1927, described as "literally Transcribed with Introduction and Notes". It is useful for its comparison with the ordinances of other foundations, especially Whitgift's, shewing how Abbot drew from other sources, modifying what he found. The transcription, however, is far from literal. The statutes of Whitgift's hospital in Croydon were printed in 1890, and can also be found in Ducarel 1790 pp 135-48.

16. Perhaps he thought that the Mores of Loseley could look after the poor of that part of St Nicolas' parish.

17. Abbot directed that after his death a prayer should be said daily in the chapel in thanksgiving for himself and Sir Nicholas Kempe. The form of the prayer was not given, and it may have fallen to William Laud, as Archbishop, to compose it. (Laud received a copy of the statutes in April 1634.) The prayer has been revised several times, most recently in 1986.

18. A problem with Highlands had to be settled, a lease dated 4 May 1617 for a thousand years from 1632. The hospital archives contain a very notable collection of documents relating to these and other properties, many of them with seals intact. The oldest dated writing is of

8 November 1370, in the Highlands series, which is the longest, with forty-one items from before the end of the reign of Henry VIII. A list was published in Powell and Jenkinson 1930 pp 50-84, in which, however, the earlier Charlwood documents, 1542-1652, are not included.

19. There was some uncertainty about Abbot's intentions for the fuel endowment. The land at St Catherine's bought from Bromfield is listed in statute 28, 17 August 1629, but in the deed of endowment, 11 July 1629, Brooklands in Chiddingfold is named. This comparatively small part of the funding of the hospital was not resolved until 1632, with the purchase of West Wantley farm.

20. Whitgift regulated important things carefully, but he did not fuss over little details, which Abbot could not leave alone.

21. The child was buried two days later. The master had two sons called Richard. The first died in his second year; the second, born in 1587, was the father of the baby Thomas, and of an older son Richard, born in 1619, whose baptism is not recorded in Guildford, who became a fellow of Corpus Christi College Oxford in 1648.

22. The cost of the hospital and of the manufacture building is not known, as no record of the larger disbursements by the Archbishop has yet been found.

Abbot's Hospital Guildford

THREE
THE MANUFACTURE AND THE SCHOOL

The Archbishop's first intention was to found a charity that would in some measure restore prosperity to the cloth industry in Guildford, and that was the subject of his letter to the Mayor in December 1614. He soon decided to found the hospital, but did not give up his earlier intention, and a large building was erected behind the hospital, west of the garden. Chapter 26 of the hospital statutes gives directions for the management of this "manufacture". In 1627 Abbot bought from Thomas Polesden a farm of about sixty-five acres called Testers (later called Tifters) at Charlwood, Surrey. He paid £680 for it, and it yielded £40 annually. In 1629 he bought land at Burstow and at Horne, Surrey, from Mr Bishe, for £1120, yielding £60.[1] This land amounted to two hundred and twenty-five acres. The ledger and the other records of the manufacture were to be kept in the evidence house of the hospital, under the custody of the master and other key-keepers, but control was in the hands of the Mayor and his brethren, as trustees, who were to employ a clerk for twenty shillings a year. Each year, on 10 or 11 November, a decision was to be made about the nature of the work to be undertaken in the following year. Care was to be taken that the finances of the hospital and the manufacture were not "mingled".

In 1627 Richard Brigham was in Guildford, working at setting up the manufacture. In 1629 the stable was altered to make more room for the workmen. (The stalls for the horses were moved into the hospital, presumably into the cellars under the north block.) Money was left with Richard Abbot to pay for this work and £50 was handed over in the winter of 1629-30. Very soon after his arrival Jasper Yardley caused the scheme to be put into operation. It was decided that linen should be made, probably so that there should be no interference with other businesses in the town, for the woollen industry was already suffering from the lack of oversea trade. In April 1630 Yardley paid £20 to rent some land and to grow flax and hemp. In August he paid £10 for harvesting the crop. An instructor was engaged, and the industry was started, and some linen was produced. In August 1631 cloths were made for the two long tables in the common hall of the hospital.

In July 1632 George Abbot made his will. He commended the manufacture to the Mayor and borough dignitaries, and also laid down that his gift of £100 in 1614 was to be used for loans to four poor tradesmen for two or three years at the most, to aid them in their work. If a borrower died, the money was to be returned within three months. So, when he died in 1633, Abbot knew that both parts of his foundation, the hospital and the manufacture, were in operation, fully endowed to the extent that he considered necessary.

The weaving of linen did not prove a successful enterprise, and there is no reference to it after 1633. The running of the workshop, and the employment of weavers, cost more than the income from rents, and there was little demand for what was produced. Furthermore, there was resentment in the town against the manufacture workers, who appeared to be a privileged group. After the Archbishop's death, the trustees took advantage of the discretion given in the statutes, and decided to change to the making of woollen cloth. Four years' rent accumulated while no work was being done, and some of this was spent on converting the workshop to its new use. The manufacture opened again in 1638, and in November the brothers and sisters of the hospital were provided with gowns made from cloth woven there. A garden north of the hospital was rented for 1s. 8d a year, and there were placed two racks, or tenter frames, where the cloth was held firmly while it dried after dyeing. Yardley, the master of the hospital encouraged this change. His successor, in 1639, was Henry Snelling, a clothworker, and he gave knowledgeable support. He bought a ledger for 2s. 6d, and took the annual clerk's fee of £1 for his work, but after his death in 1643, there was another decline, and work stopped in 1644. In July that year, Maurice Abbot, the founder's nephew and executor, wrote to the Mayor, "I believe if my Lord were alive himself he would dispense with his owne Rules, in this case, whn the Towne standes so much in neede". Nonetheless the looms were still there, and another attempt was made, in 1647. A deputation, including the Mayor, John Martin, and the master, went to London to discuss it with Maurice Abbot. A loan of £400 was made without security to John Stanton "for the ymployinge of the Manufacture worke". The master of the manufacture until his death in 1650 was Richard Woodyer, who also acted for the Mayor in the business of Sir Richard Weston's development of the Wey Navigation. He was succeeded in both offices by Richard Scotcher. Woodyer and Scotcher had worked in the manufacture when Yardley and Snelling were masters of the hospital. The manufacture ran until 1655, and then foundered, with little return for the outlay. During this time some of the income was used for the benefit of the poor. Between 1648 and 1655, grants were made amounting to £130, and loans of £501. 10s.[2]

It was clear that Abbot's plan would not succeed, and that his endowment was not effectually helping the young and poor to be set up in the cloth industry. It was badly conceived. If business was good at the manufacture, the endowment was not strictly necessary; if business flagged, then the endowment provided a subsidy which put other clothworkers in the town at a disadvantage.

A judgment was sought in the Court of Chancery, and delivered on 3 July 1656. With immediate effect the income of the manufacture endowment was to be used to make small annual grants to ten or more poor honest workmen in the town. The rents were to be collected from the farms and handed over to the Mayor. The two years' revenue received since work stopped was also to be distributed in this way. Grants were begun on 13 August. The division of the £200 was: Holy Trinity parish, eleven grants to the total of £75; St Mary's parish, thirteen grants amounting to £91.13.4d; St Nicolas' parish, five grants amounting to £33.6.8d. Until 1662 the grants were usually of £5. In 1663 they were £2.10s, so that the beneficiaries could be doubled in number. From 1664 the grants were of variable sums. Abbot's original gift of £100, to be used for loans, had not been properly accounted, and was considered to be absorbed and fulfilled in this Chancery scheme.

The Manufacture and The School

In 1658 it was decided that the old stable was not likely to be needed for workmen again, and it was altered and restored to the use of the hospital for its original purpose. The cost, £63.16.6½d, was met from the manufacture funds.[3]

The Chancery scheme gave no direction for the use of the manufacture building. It was kept in repair, and later in the century it met a new need. At some time between 1660 and 1673 a union workhouse for the three Guildford parishes was built against the north end wall of the manufacture so that its doorway[4] led straight into the new premises. The workhouse was a plain brick structure of three storeys and an attic floor, similar in style to the manufacture,[5] whose length it nearly doubled. The older building came to be used as the infirmary for the workhouse, and to be known as the "lower hospital". Although it was used by the parishes, repairs were still paid for from the manufacture income. No rent appears to have been paid for the use of the building until the eighteen-twenties, when St Mary's and St Nicolas' parishes each paid two guineas a year for a room. Holy Trinity paid nothing. When Samuel Robinson became master of the hospital in 1824, he decided that the occupants of the Holy Trinity rooms were objectionable, and that Holy Trinity should pay fourteen years of rent arrears at £10 a year. After a second warning, Holy Trinity removed the residents, but did not pay the money claimed. St Mary's and St Nicolas' wished to have the use of the vacated rooms for ten guineas a year, but it was decided that all three parishes should continue to use the building, and pay a total rent of £12. The first payment was due at Michaelmas 1825, and was made the following July.

For over a century the grants to the poor were made, and became virtually a small dole. At the end of the seventeenth century they were as little as ten shillings, or even five, but as the eighteenth century passed, sums of between one and three pounds were given. In 1705 the Mayor and magistrates agreed that no payments should be made to "any Foreigners or other person or persons who had not obtained a legall settlement within this Towne & Corporation" by 25 March 1695.

A major increase in the hospital's establishment came in 1785, by an order in Chancery of 14 December, putting into effect the gift of Alderman Thomas Jackman.[6] One result of this was the diversion of half the manufacture endowment to the hospital, leaving only £50 for the annual distribution to the poor. By the eighteen-thirties this was done in Christmas week, eighty to one hundred recipients being chosen by the Mayor and aldermen from the old borough part of the three town parishes.

These arrangements continued until the changes of the age of reform. A consequence of the Poor Law Amendment Act of 1834 was the setting up of the Guildford Board of Guardians in 1836, and the building of a new workhouse to serve an enlarged union of parishes. It opened in Chalky Lane, renamed Union Lane,[7] in July 1838. The inmates of the lower hospital evidently moved away before that, as the last rent was received in July 1836. The building was leased to Christopher Fry from 25 March 1837, for a quarterly rent of £6. Soon the lease was varied, and the old manufacture was converted into four tenements or cottages, to bring in a rent of half a crown a week each. This was taken by the hospital, but it should have been shared with the Mayor, to increase the distribution to the poor. The old workhouse was sold by the Board of Guardians in May 1837, and was soon divided into tenements. The northernmost part of it had become the Crown Inn at least by 1862.[8]

Further reform was approaching. Surveys were made of all charitable institutions, and the information that was collected was used as the basis for proposals to make the foundations more suited to the needs of the times.[9] A decree of Chancery of 10 March 1852 ordered an enquiry into the manufacture charity. The payments to the poor were made for the last time in that year. While the enquiries were being made, the suggestion arose that the endowment should be combined with that of the Bluecoat School, founded under the will of Thomas Baker, who died in 1584. Since 1762 this school had met in the tower of Holy Trinity Church. The capital endowment of the Bluecoat School was £840, which brought in an income of £24.1.6d. The master of the hospital, George Russell, noted on 4 January 1855 that Charlwood and Burstow farms, and the four cottages behind the hospital were given up to the commissioner, and on 14 May he surrendered the cottage keys. Russell provided a certificate of the manufacture finances, dated 15 June 1855, and that was used as the basis for the scheme for the new trust set up by Chancery order of 17 July that same year, founding the Archbishop Abbot's School.[10]

The basis of the financial arrangements that had to be made was the fact that Abbot had left an income of £200 for the hospital and £100 for the manufacture. This proportion of two : one was used in the division of the endowments. At first part of the school's income was a charge on the hospital's revenues. Rents from the farms were divided, and also the interest from bank stock. The capital to be considered was £2984.15.6d. The school was paid the three per cent interest of one third of this sum, the first payment, £14.18.6d, being made on 23 May 1856. The initial annual income of the school may be summarised:

rents from the manufacture farms, Charlwood and Burstow, including house	100.	0.	0d
one third of the rents from the properties acquired by the hospital since its foundation	31.	0.	0d
one third of the interest from bank stock	29.	16.	11d
	£160.	16.	11d

From this was deducted an annual charge of £8 to be paid to an out sister, Mrs Jelly, until she succeeded to a vacancy in the hospital. The old endowment of the Bluecoat School was entirely used up in the payment of legal costs and the alterations to the building to make it suitable for a school.

The Order in Chancery of 17 July 1855 vested the new school in named trustees: Thomas Ludham, Rector of Holy Trinity and St Mary since 1851, Samuel Paynter, Rector of Stoke since 1831, William Henley Pearson, Rector of St Nicolas' since 1837, Ross

Donnelly Mangles, MP for Guildford since 1841, William Edward Elkins, James Stedman, Thomas Haydon, William Newland, Cassteels Cooper, Joseph Weale, John Ryde Cooke and Samuel Haydon.

The trustees met for the first time on 7 October 1856, with Ludham in the chair for that day. One of their first acts was to insure the school for £500. The building was adapted for its new use by John Pearce, following plans drawn up by the architect Henry Clutton. There were two classrooms and a house for the head master. The cost of the work, including fees, was £726.9.8d. The legal fees for the promotion of the scheme amounted to £747.6.8d (Archbishop of Canterbury £54.4.8d, school and hospital £273.13.lld, Attorney General £418.18.1d). Together, the alterations and costs exceeded the sum available from the Bluecoat endowment (£840, with £63.13.8d accumulated income) and a balance in the manufacture funds of £210.12.10. Timber was sold at Burstow and Charlwood for £327.6.6d to meet most of the deficit, and some delay was allowed in paying the Attorney General's fee.

On 13 October the trustees appointed Robert Lidgate as the first head master, and Sampson Court was chosen as second master on 15 December. The boys were all admitted by the trustees. Thirty, all resident in the borough of Guildford, were to be educated without charge, and were known as Baker's boys. On 15 December forty-four paying boys were selected. They were permitted by the scheme, "being of good character, and not affected with any infectious or offensive disease". Their quarterly fees were two shillings for the sons of labourers and artisans. For others the fees began at five shillings for those below eight years, rising to ten shillings (8 - 10), fifteen shillings (10 - 12) and twenty shillings (over 12). Through the school's history, boys were regularly promoted from the paying list to be Baker's boys. Boys living outside the borough could be admitted to the school only if there was room. The academic expenditure was not expected to be large. The head's salary was £80 for the year, and his assistant was paid £50. Prizes might cost £5, and each year the school was to be examined by a graduate of an English university, with no local connexions. His fee was not to exceed five guineas. Books, paper, pencils and pens were to be provided by the parents, though the trustees were allowed to supply them when there was need.

The school opened early in 1857, with little to relieve the bareness of the old building. Gas had been laid on in 1856 in readiness, and forms were provided for the pupils' use in January. The head was to provide maps and unspecified apparatus. The curriculum comprised the principles of the Christian religion, reading, writing, arithmetic, general English literature and composition, sacred and profane history, geography, book-keeping, land surveying, drawing and the principles of design - and anything further that the trustees might add. Daily morning prayers and religious instruction were to be according to the rites and principles of the Church of England, but with a right of withdrawal for parents who objected to this.

School life seems to have been uneventful, and the trustees did not have any serious problems to deal with - until they found it necessary to reprimand the head master in October 1862, when they discovered that he had been absent for three consecutive days so that he could watch cricket. Lidgate resigned early in 1864, and was replaced by James Macfarland, appointed on 2 March, who remained until the end of 1887. The trustees were concerned about ventilation, and about bad smells from the Crown Inn. In October 1862 they asked the Charity Commission for access through the hospital grounds, and for permission to use part of the garden as a playground. In April they raised the matter again with the newly constituted board of Governors of the hospital. It was agreed that part of the western wall of the hospital garden should be replaced with railings, but access and playground space were not approved.

In April 1865 the trustees met to consider a complaint against the second master, Rouse, accused by a parent of assault on his son. Rouse remained in his appointment, but a policy was laid down, surprisingly modern in its detail: "(1) that no corporal punishment should be given by anyone other than the head master. (2) and that such punishment should be confined when such chastisement might be thought necessary, to that inflicted with the cane, and should be administered at some interval after the offence."

The division of income with the hospital was soon found unsatisfactory by both bodies. A Charity Commission report in 1860 recommended that the estates should be divided in the historic proportion 2:1, in the hospital's favour. In March 1862 the Commission indicated that Robert Clutton was appointed to survey the land for fair division. He refused, and the Commission accepted the Governors' suggestion of Job Smallpeice. Correspondence continued into 1865. At one point the Governors proposed that they should buy out the school's share of the endowment property, but this was not followed up. The need for a playground was pressed by the trustees, and the yard between the school and the stable, used as a drying ground, was suggested, and both bodies agreed that it should be included in the school's share. This was approved by the Commission in October 1862, but in the end it was not transferred. Instead it was agreed, in May 1864, that the yard should be rented by the school for a yearly payment on one pound.[11]

On 5 April 1865, a joint meeting of Governors and trustees accepted the apportionment worked out by Smallpeice. The Commission suggested that a formal instrument of the award should be drawn up. This was agreed, and it was completed on 29 September 1866. The business was concluded on 2 January 1867. The hospital was to retain Tankerleys farm at Dorking, and Woolpits farm at Ewhurst except for Dean Hurst field. The school acquired Salthurst farm at Ewhurst, and Dean Hurst field, as well at three tenements and gardens, a barn and a yard called Martin's Plat, part of Merrow farm. All this was added to the school's endowment farms at Burstow and Charlwood. There had already been a change at Burstow. In February 1865, the Charity Commission approved the exchange of eighty-four acres of the estate with the slightly larger part of Rookery farm.

The Manufacture and The School

The management of the estates took up much of the trustees' meeting time, as it always had in the affairs of the hospital. Farm buildings needed to be repaired, and there were sometimes wrangles with neighbours over boundaries. Money for repairs was usually raised by the sale of timber. In 1876 a further twenty-one acres was bought at Burstow, adjacent to Rookery farm, for £1133.13s, £333.13s of which was raised by selling timber. At the same time Salthurst farm was sold, for £900.

Improvement of the school building was considered in 1869, when the local architect W.G. Lower was asked for plans and estimates for a scheme to give more room and better ventilation. Nothing was done at the time, and when the stable fell vacant in 1871 the Governors offered it for use as a classroom for a rent of £7 a year, the cost of alterations to be borne by the trustees. W.G. Lower's estimate for the necessary work was £169, which the trustees considered too much, so that idea was given up. In January 1872 Lower produced plans for a classroom on the attic floor. The Charity Commission gave approval, on condition that the greatest possible height was achieved - between fourteen and fifteen feet. This was done by removing the ceiling in the northern section of the top floor. The work was completed for £323.17.6d, by G. Strudwick. Lower's fee was £22.14.6d. While the workmen were there, an iron pipe and a drinking tap for the boys were installed.[12] The Governors of the hospital allowed the school to use the dining hall for a few weeks while the builders were at work.

After the improvements, the insurance cover was raised to £1500 (school £800, house £500, school fittings £200). Little is known of the school's equipment, as there are few references in the trustees' minutes. In 1870, Mr John Nealds, one of the trustees, and a generous supporter of the school, gave "a Galvanic Battery and Philosophical Apparatus". In 1874 new maps were bought for £4.8.6d, and in 1875 a large black slate for £3. In 1881 the Charity Commission approved increased salaries. The head master was to be paid £100 and the assistant £75. In addition a pupil teacher might be appointed for £6.

In the 1880s, when the school had established its place in the town, there was a threat to its existence. In 1883 the Charity Commission, acting with powers acquired following the Endowed Schools Act 1869, began to make suggestions for the revival of the Grammar School, and for the restoration of its dilapidated buildings. In 1884 there was a proposal that Archbishop Abbot's School should be amalgamated with the Grammar School. The trustees rejected this at their meeting on 5 August, and for a while maintained their opposition, though they began to waver under much pressure. A local tailor, and old boy of the school, P.G. Palmer, who was later to become master of the hospital, organised a petition to save Archbishop Abbot's School as a separate institution. The argument was that the free Baker's places were a benefit to the poor that would disappear if the endowments were absorbed into those of the Grammar School. Opposition to the amalgamation was also strong from those who saw it as a threat to the proper development of the Grammar School, and late in 1887 it was learnt that the proposal had been withdrawn.[13] It was then that Macfarland retired, to be replaced by Arthur Slater, who had been head master of St Nicolas' School. A Royal Commission report in 1895 confirmed that there was a place for both schools, considering that Archbishop Abbot's School fulfilled the function of a higher grade elementary school. It recommended that girls should be admitted, but this step was never taken.[14]

Soon after the continued life of the school was assured, an opportunity arose for expansion. On 15 February 1889 the clerk reported to the trustees that the adjoining property, the former workhouse. was about to be sold. It had been bought by William Simmonds of Farnham in 1867, and leased in 1870 to Thomas Taunton, the brewer of the Cannon Brewery, Guildford. C.H. Master, who was briefly in partnership with Taunton in 1873, bought the business from him, and when the old workhouse was sold, he bought that part of it which was the Crown Inn. The school trustees quickly decided to bid for the house that formed the southern part of the property, and secured it on 2 April for £430.[15] The Charity Commission approved the purchase, and allowed the trustees to sell land at Merrow to Lord Onslow for £419.10s. Timber at Charlwood had been sold for £54.12s in 1888, and a bigger sale of timber at Charlwood and Burstow (£286) followed in 1891. The newly acquired house had a sitting tenant, but he was allowed to remain there until Lady Day 1891, for an annual rent of £18.

On 6 January 1891 W.G. Lower was instructed to make proposals for converting the house for use by the school. He estimated that his scheme would cost £800. In April the approval of the Charity Commission for Lower's plans was reported, and tenders were invited. They were high, and that of Mitchells Bros was chosen, at £975, which rose to £1275 during the work.[16] The Charity Commission gave permission for £750 consols to be sold, towards the cost of the new structure, which took the form of a brick tower, entered from the west, with a two-tiered oriel window above the doorway, and small turrets at the corners of the parapet.

In 1896, Slater was replaced as head master by Richard Cooke, who had been second master since 1886. Cooke remained in office for over thirty years, and for the whole of that time struggled to maintain reasonable standards without an adequate income. In 1898 the endowment income was only a little over £200. Fees were still at the 1857 level (and were not raised until 1909), and the Baker's boys were educated free, according to the scheme. An improvement came with the sale of the farms. The Rookery at Burstow was sold in 1918 for £4000, and Tifters at Charlwood in 1919 for £2100. The proceeds were invested in 4 per cent funding stock. All that remained of the ancient endowment was little more than an acre at Horne, bringing in fifteen shillings in rent, and for which no purchaser was found.

There seems to have been little formal business between the school and the hospital, after the apportionment of property had been settled. In October 1917, the Governors approved the use of the hospital cellars for a refuge for the boys "in case of a Daylight Air Raid". Early in 1919 the trustees were sharply reminded of arrears in the payment of the playground rent, for which the Governors "did not see their way to compromise".

The Manufacture and The School

Almost at the end of Cooke's years as head master, in October 1927, the decision was made by the trustees, "to abolish slates at the School and introduce paper instead". In the following year, Cooke was succeeded by the Reverend Clifford Fernihough, a graduate of Manchester, with a master's degree in education.[17] Additional room was secured when the stable was at last acquired. The hospital Governors offered it in 1928, and the trustees suggested a rent of £15. The Governors fixed it at £12.10s, and the school occupied it from early in 1929.

After the founding of the diocese of Guildford, in 1927, when Holy Trinity Church was used as the cathedral, an arrangement was made for educating ten choristers at Archbishop Abbot's School, and their fees were paid by the church council from 1928. This small increase in income made little difference to the plight of the school. In 1930 the endowment income from investments was £373.10.2d. (No rent had been received from Horne since 1927, when it had risen to £3.) Fees amounted to £889.8.11.d, and subscriptions brought in another £371, resulting in an income of £1633.19.1d. This was not nearly enough to run an efficient school for over one hundred boys. Appeals to the public, the County Council, the diocese and to some city companies all failed to produce either a capital sum or an assured income, and discussions began to include the possibility of closing the school. In February 1932 it was agreed that no new boys should be admitted, and on 18 August the decision was taken to close the school. It was marked by a Latin service in Holy Trinity on 22 December, and the boys were dispersed among other schools, where for some of them fees were paid by the trustees.

In July 1932 the trustees decided that George Abbot's benefaction to the workers of the town should take yet another form, and the approval of the Charity Commission was secured. A new trust was set up by a scheme dated 20 April 1933, establishing the Archbishop Abbot's Exhibition Foundation. There were to be seven trustees, though to begin with the number was larger, as all the existing trustees of the school were named as life trustees of the foundation – the Venerable Lionel Edward Blackburne, Archdeacon of Surrey, Sir Claude Fraser de la Fosse, the Reverend Thomas William Graham, Rector of Stoke, Thomas Gatton Swayne, Harry George Herbert, John Marina Sumpster, Harry Shepard Higlett, Harvey Mansbridge Lunn and Arthur Lindsay Kelly. These were to be replaced by co-opting, but not before the number fell below four, those co-opted to serve for five years. The other three trustees were to be appointed by the Borough Council for three years, the County Council for a term until replaced, and the Bishop of Guildford for three years. They chose Alderman Charles Thomas Bateman, Percy Thomas Fairbrother and Arthur John Bradford Green, head master of the Grammar School, respectively.

The revenues of the foundation, when costs of administration had been met, were to be used to provide exhibitions to be awarded to boys living in the borough of Guildford, to assist them "to attend schools, universities or other institutions or classes, for purposes of education other than elementary". The money, which might be called Baker

Exhibitions, could be used for fees, maintenance, travel or meals. Any surplus income was to be added to the capital.

A use had to be found for the school building, to produce an income. There was a suggestion, raised by the Borough Council, that the Council should use it for a junior technical school. The Surrey County Council thought of opening a junior commercial school there, and the trustees offered a three-year lease for an annual rent of £50. Neither of these proposals was followed up. The Young Men's Christian Association shewed interest, but decided that the building was not large enough for their purposes. In 1933 Clark's College Limited became the tenants of the trustees, and a twenty-one-year lease was signed on 14 December, some time after the company's school had moved into the building.[18] The annual rent was £175, but it was not received by the foundation for long. The Governors of the hospital approached the trustees with the request to buy the building. Agreement was reached in October 1933, and a year later, on 22 October 1934, the sale price of £4000 was received.[19] After that, the Old Cloth Hall, as it came to be called, was part of the history of the hospital.

In 1936, the land at Horne was sold for £100 - the last of the original manufacture endowment to be disposed of. Like the proceeds of the sale of the building, the money was added to the capital investment, and placed in 3% local loans stock.

As years passed, there were insufficient applications for Baker exhibitions for all the income to be used. On 7 May 1959, the trustees resolved to seek a widening of the scope of the foundation, both in the area of benefit and the purposes for which grants could be given. The variation of the scheme was sealed on 25 April 1960. The borough of Godalming, the urban district of Haslemere, and the rural districts of Guildford and Hambledon were added to the area of benefit, and grants could be made for the additional purposes of buying clothing, books or other equipment "to enable beneficiaries on leaving school, a university or any other educational establishment to prepare for, or to assist their entry into, a profession, trade or calling"; also for educational travel abroad, "for recreation and social and physical training, including the provision of coaching in athletics, sports and games", and for the study of music or other arts. Exhibitions could also be given to boys without residential qualifications but who had attended or were to attend a school within the borough of Guildford as constituted then. The ages of beneficiaries were to be between eleven and twenty-five. By the Local Government Act, 1972, the borough of Guildford was made much larger from 1 April 1974, and other changes were made to the area of benefit, which is now defined as "the area administered by the Guildford Borough Council or the Waverley Borough Council (except that part of Waverley formerly within the Urban District of Farnham)".[20]

The Charity Commission authorised a further variation of the scheme on 15 May 1989. The range of benefit was cautiously extended: "the expression 'beneficiaries' means persons with a preference for males".

The Manufacture and The School

1. Both Charlwood and Burstow parishes were peculiars, under the jurisdiction of the Archbishop of Canterbury, so his agents were well placed to purchase land as it became available.

2. Some of the accumulated funds of the manufacture were lent to the churchwardens of Holy Trinity to repair houses in their possession, £30 in 1650 and £70 in 1651. Repayment, without interest, was completed in 1676. During the meeting with Maurice Abbot, a loan of £400 was agreed to the mayor for the Poyle estate, for the repair of the town mills, which had been given by Henry Smith in 1643 for the benefit of the poor of the town.

3. P.G. Palmer suggested that part of this much altered building, now the caretaker's cottage, had survived from the stable of the Half Moon inn, which occupied the western part of the hospital site until it was bought by Abbot in 1618. This is not probable. The style of the building, with its formal east elevation with pilasters, and the amount of money spent, suggest that the 1658 work was a virtual replacement, designed to match the hospital suitably. Mr Matthew Alexander and Mr Charles Brooking kindly inspected the cottage on 8 October 1987, and came to this conclusion.

4. The doorway had opened onto the clear space known as the north town ditch, where North Street is now.

5. The only picture that is available is the water colour by John Hassell

6. This will be described in chapter 4.

7. This is now Warren Road. The workhouse became part of the Guildford Union Infirmary in 1896, later called Warren Road Hospital, and more recently St Luke's Hospital. The story is given in Davies 1982, pp 53-57, 64-67.

8. There is a reference to the "Crown tap", 1839-41.

9. This will be dealt with in chapter 4. The report on the hospital and manufacture can be found in Smith 1839, pp 881-891.

10. For the history of Archbishop Abbot's School, and the school establishments that lay behind it, see Barlow 1924, and Green 1954, pp 1-7.

11. The ground was used, for the same rent, until the school closed. The first payment was not made until 1870 - six years in arrears.

12. The trustees also gave permission for the head master's bedroom to be painted and papered. The wallpaper was not to cost more than 2d a yard.

13. An account of the controversy, more from the point of view of the Grammar School, will be found in Sturley 1980, pp 103-105.

14. For the report and recommendations, with comparative figures for Surrey schools, see Headlam 1895, pp 7, 9-10. In a report published in 1868, an earlier commission had suggested that the Archbishop Abbot's School might become the preparatory department of the Grammar School. A similar suggestion was to be made in 1931.

15. Information about the Crown Inn was kindly supplied by Mr D.M. Sturley whose *The Breweries and Public Houses of Guildford* (Guildford 1990) gives details of all the town's

licensed premises. The Crown was sold to the Mayor and corporation in 1907, and demolished for road-widening.

16. Lower's design was modified following a survey by E. Christian, known in Guildford as the architect of Christ Church, and for executing S.S. Teulon's designs for the rebuilt St Nicolas'. Christian's fee was two guineas. Mitchells had a difficult task. The Crown had to be kept standing while the house was demolished, for they had been part of one building. Furthermore, the north wall of the tower had to be built from the inside.

17. Fernihough was ordained deacon only in 1928, and was associated with Holy Trinity until 1930, and then with Farnham. From his ordination as priest in 1931 he assisted at St Saviour's.

18. Clark's College, founded in 1880, opened a school in St Nicolas' House, Portsmouth Road Guildford, in 1921.

19. The costs of the transaction (vendors' £52.5s, purchasers' £82.9s) were borne by the Governors of the hospital.

20. The records of the Archbishop Abbot's School are now deposited in the Guildford Muniment Room. I am grateful to Mr Colin Fullagar for making them available in their previous place, and for information concerning the Exhibition Foundation.

FOUR
THE HOSPITAL 1633 - 1846

Jasper Yardley continued as master of the hospital for nearly six years after the founder's death. Until shortly before his own death, he kept the ledger meticulously, and both the community and the property were well cared for. On 29 October 1633, George Abbot's birthday, he took an inventory of the contents of the hospital.[1] All that was provided in the rooms of the brothers and sisters were "halfe headed Bedsteds". Some of the equipment had been acquired by Yardley already, including the "great brasse pott" weighing 42 pounds, bought in 1631, with its handles, for £1.12s.[2] In the treasury, the upper room in the tower, were kept the documents relating to the hospital lands, the charter and the statutes, as well as the common seal, of brass. There was also an amount of silver, "Two silver Boles, a great & a lesse, Two silver Saultes a great & a less, & two dozen of silver Spoones, one lesse, the other greater".[3]

The hospital bell was probably hung outside the north-east turret at first, and then was rehung inside when the turrets were completed. The cost of rehanging was one shilling. New fittings of iron, with a pulley, were added in 1636-7, for 3/2d. Bellropes lasted only about two years. A new cord in 1630 cost ten pence, but better quality ones were used afterwards.

Examples of expenditure include two baskets for carrying coal, 1/10d; a shovel, 1/1d; a tub for fetching beer, 1/6d; eight pewter dishes, 22/-d; the labour for making three forms for the gate, 7d. These were presumably made from spare pieces of wood, and provided so that the residents could watch the world go by. Some money had to be spent on the garden. Shears were ground and mended, 1/-d; a mole was killed, 4d; "for getting the garden rake out of the well tht fell in before I came", 6d. Occasionally a gardener was employed for a day, 8d. Cloth for making gowns for the residents was bought every two years. That was as long as they would last, if used as their outer garment all the time. While Abbot was alive, he controlled admission to the hospital. Former servants did not have to be over sixty years of age, by chapter 5 of the statutes. On 15 April 1632 James Berriman was admitted, aged 53, but he died within a month. Other retired servants were admitted for a number of years, and also some who claimed to be founder's kin. The first vacancy after the founder's death was filled by the mayor, William Hill, on 6 June 1634, who chose Ann Hillar. Thereafter nominations were made by the master and mayor alternately, according to the statutes.

Yardley delivered a copy of the hospital statutes to Laud, as the new visitor. It may well have been the Archbishop who then provided the form for the daily commemoration of the founder.

Abbot's Hospital Guildford

As George Abbot's affairs were settled, three important gifts were made to the hospital by Sir Morris from Croydon. The portrait of the founder that hangs in the boardroom is believed to have been painted by a Flemish artist in 1623. Some months after Abbot's funeral, his hatchment was fetched, and put into the chapel, and that was followed by the portrait of Sir Nicholas Kempe, now in the boardroom, painted by Paul van Somer.

Richard Abbot, a grocer, and the son of the Archbishop's eldest brother, the first master of the hospital, was perhaps offended at the dissatisfaction with his father's management, and he may have been envious of the trust placed in Sir Morris. After the founder's death, he claimed to be his heir, and in particular laid claim to West Wantley farm. On 6 February 1636, Sir Morris Abbot and his son Maurice, with the master and the brethren, executed a deed acknowledging Richard as heir, and his ownership of West Wantley farm. In reponse to this, Richard placed a yearly charge of £12.10s on the estate, and a covenant to this effect was included in the conditions of sale when it was bought from Richard by Gregory Haines of Shere, in June 1642. The covenant remains, and the payment of £12.50p is still made to the hospital.

One of the founder's fussy rules was the order in chapter 28 of the statutes that a secret fund of £100 should be accumulated, and "carefully kept in golde against time of extremitie, and none of it to be taken out without greate cause". Yardley achieved this in 1633, and the money was locked up in the treasury. Successive masters, on their appointment, took note of what came to be called the old gold - but it depreciated in value. This scheme shews the mind of George Abbot, almost certainly acting without the city-wise advice of his brother Morris.

Jasper Yardley died on 31 May 1639, aged only 59, and was buried at Holy Trinity Church. In his will he left £5 to the hospital for buying coal, and made bequests to the parishes of Guildford and Croydon, and several London parishes. In Yardley's place, on the day he died, Henry Snelling was chosen as master. He was a clothworker, and his election was the first to be conducted according to the statutes. Out of his own working experience he did what he could to help the manufacture prosper, and started a separate ledger for its accounts. New gowns were needed in 1641. Snelling bought the cloth from the manufacture (113 yards for £25.8.6d) and paid £1.11.6d for them to be made up there.

Repairs and improvements continued. In 1643, sand and flints were bought, "for pitching the court", at a total cost of £7.4.0½d. Two shillings bought a blackjack for drawing beer, and an iron spit for roasting meat on gaudy days. In 1641 a long wicker brush was bought for 2½d, "to sweepe downe the Cobwebs in the Chappell". A little ladder was bought for sixpence, for pruning trees, in 1639. In 1640 Snelling spent 1/3d on three dozen gooseberry bushes and one dozen rose trees. In 1644, sixpence was spent on beating the walnuts from the tree. By this time the daily rate for a gardener had risen to 1/6d; his assistant received 1/2d.

The Hospital 1633-1864

While Snelling was master, England moved towards civil war, which began when King Charles raised his standard at Nottingham in August 1642. References in the hospital ledger to gates and locks shew anxiety about security. The balance of power in the county was a matter of pressing concern for Guildford.[4] The High Sherriff of Surrey, Sir John Denham of Egham, raised a loan for the King, and the hospital was compelled to pay £100 on 9 November 1642. The following day the parliamentary garrison of Farnham Castle was evicted, and marched through Guildford to Kingston. It was expected that they would soon return and be billeted in the town. The parliamentary troops did return, under Sir William Waller. They stayed for two days, and then went on to recover Farnham Castle on 1 December.

The hospital began to pay subsidies for the militia in 1643. There was fear for the safety of the money that had accumulated in the treasury, and it was decided to send it to London. A wooden box was made (4/4d), with a cord "to encoyle it"(4d), and the coins were packed into four linen bags (1/-).[5] The total was £580 (hospital £399.1.1d, manufacture £180.18.11d). William Smallpeice was paid five shillings for the journey and the risk, and the box was entrusted to Mr Leigh, a linen draper of Fish Street Hill, on 7 November.

During these exciting times, Henry Snelling died, on 18 November 1643, and was buried at St Mary's. On the day of Snelling's death, Thomas Smith, a maltster, was chosen to succeed him.

Smith was master for less than nine months, and worked under great difficulties. He had no reserves of money, and rents from the farms were slow coming in. The times were confused, and he had no superior to turn to for authoritative advice. The Visitor, Archbishop Laud, had been imprisoned since December 1640, and even more significantly, Sir Morris Abbot had died late in 1642. A loan to Sir Richard Onslow was recorded on 7 June 1644, £60 for the use of Parliament. Onslow was supposed to raise it from the town, but failed, and turned to the hospital and manufacture for help. Later the borough accepted liability, but never paid the money back.

Changes in the Church reached the hospital while Smith was master. The Rector of Holy Trinity, Thomas Wall, was dispossessed on 6 June 1644, and replaced by a succession of preaching ministers, who, it may be assumed, did not use the Book of Common Prayer.[6] The high church Rector of St Nicolas', Dr Nicholas Andrewes, had been ejected in 1643. At St Mary's, William Kay, who had been Rector since 1605, managed to comply with changed ways, and stayed there until his death in 1650.

Thomas Smith died on 2 August 1644. The next day Henry Horner, a barber-surgeon, was chosen to be master in his place. It was not an easy task, as money was always short, and war loans continued to be exacted. In the seven half-yearly accounts, Lady day 1644 to Lady day 1647, farm rents amounted to £666.5s, from which £11.6.8d was withheld by the tenants to pay for repairs. Taxation and the charge for quartering soldiers reduced the hospital's income, so that for that period there was a deficit of £203.5.9½d, to which rising costs also contributed. Economy was necessary. New gowns were made when needed, but there was also an item in the accounts for 1648 - "Payd for scouring of 2 Gownes of Deceased parties 8d". The weekly allowance of two shillings and sixpence was no longer enough for the residents to live on, and they needed the money from the almsbox, and from the fines when leases were renewed. Horner did not take his share of the fines. He visited all the farms early in his mastership, to encourage good management. He realised that timber was a valuable asset, and from his time there are frequent references in the ledgers to the trees on the farms, and to the use of the wood when they were felled, which was either sold or used for repairs to the farm properties or to the hospital.

Horner met a reminder of religious changes in his first winter. "Christmas daye fell out to be uppon the last Wednesdaye of the moneth wch was ordayned by Parliament to be kepte a fastinge daye." The celebration dinner, costing the statutory ten shillings, was held on 26th. In most of the following years, until the Restoration, 25 December was entered as "Christide", to avoid the unacceptable suffix "-mas".

The civil war approached its climax. King Charles gave himself up to the Scots at Newark on 5 May 1646, and was taken to Newcastle-on-Tyne. On 30 January 1647 the Scots handed him over to his English enemies. Before long the army advanced on London and occupied it, and there were frequent outbreaks of disorder. It was decided that the hospital's store of money would be safer in Guildford, and it was taken back in June, at a cost of 7/4d. Maurice Abbot, son of Sir Morris, a barrister of the Inner Temple, advised the Mayor and the master that the money in the chest and other available funds should be put to use, so that it could not be seized. £400 was used to restart the work of the manufacture,[7] and £400 was lent to the Mayor towards the rebuilding of the mills of the Poyle estate.[8] This was repaid to the manufacture fund in quarterly instalments of £10.

On 17 March 1649, six and a half weeks after the beheading of the King, the monarchy was abolished by Act of Parliament. On 21 August the Council of State issued a warrant to proclaim this Act, but it was not until 1651 that the hospital spent two shillings taking down the royal arms over the gateway.

Henry Horner died on 9 February 1655, and was buried at Holy Trinity the next day. His successor, chosen on the day of his death, was no stranger. John Holland, a Gloucestershire man, had been in Guildford since 1650, when he succeeded William Kay as Rector of St Mary's. Holland was a scholar, graduate and fellow of Trinity College Cambridge. Roger Percival, the minister at Holy Trinity, died in April 1654, and was followed by Holland. When the mastership of the hospital fell vacant, Holland was appointed, in accordance with chapter 2 of the statutes, which gives a certain priority to former mayors and to "the Minister who is Parson of Trinitie Church in Guilford". The statute, however, makes it plain that these privileged candidates must comply with its other provisions, to be over fifty years of age, and to be and remain single. It is very unlikely that Holland, who went up to Cambridge in 1646, was even thirty years old, and he married soon after he became master. He was master for over thirty-six years, longer by far than any other

The Hospital 1633-1864

holder of the office. It was not a bad time for the hospital, but it is difficult not to conclude that Holland was mainly moved by self-interest, and that the hospital received benefit incidentally. Holland, who abjured the Solemn League and Covenant, remained at the hospital and as Rector of St Mary's, until his death in 1691. It is not known when he was ordained as a priest, whether secretly during the interregnum, or after the restoration. Giles Thornborough received a dispensation, dated 28 June 1671, to be Rector of Holy Trinity as well as of St Nicolas', which he had held since 1660. Holland had therefore left Holy Trinity, perhaps as early as 1665. In June 1667 he became Rector of Albury, which he held until his death. The parsonage of Holy Trinity, in the south-east corner of the churchyard, was old and dilapidated, but Holland found a new home in the hospital -one of the attractions of the appointment. His wife died in December 1660, shortly after the birth of a daughter, who survived only a few weeks. In 1662 Holland married again, and five children were born, the first dying in infancy. This second wife died in 1675, shortly after the death of her ten-and-a-half year-old son. The brethren and sisters of the hospital therefore had much to interest them in the master's lodging, of a kind never visualised by the founder.

Oliver Cromwell died on 3 September 1658. His son Richard succeeded him as Lord Protector, but gave up the position on 24 May 1659, as Parliament voted him no money. In the following year Charles II was called back, and the monarchy was restored. The royal arms were put back over the hospital gate, at a cost of eighteen shillings, probably before the King visited Guildford in September 1660.

Alterations were made in the south range of the hospital. The original arrangement was that from the large ground-floor room in the south west corner a door opened to the north west turret, in which stairs led to the room above, and then stopped. A further flight of stairs began at the doorway from the "presence chamber" (now the boardroom), leading to the strongroom, or evidence house, and to the roof of the gatehouse. In 1659 Holland needed a room for a servant. He blocked the doorway from the lower room to the stairs, and put in the present doorway to the turret from the quadrangle. He had stairs made from the small room to the presence chamber level, and so completed the full flight of steps in the turret. In the same year Holland improved his own lodgings. The landing at the top of his staircase led into a large room from which steps rose to the presence chamber. A wooden screen was now made, separating most of the area into an enclosed room, leaving a corridor to the presence chamber steps. The cost of this screen was £4.5.6d and 8/6d for the lock and hinges. A porch had already been made inside the door from the quadrangle, and later on panelling was added to some of the rooms. The carpenter was Adrian van Prizzn (known as Preston).

In 1662 the bell was taken down and recast by William Eldridge of Chertsey, with $15^{1}/_{2}$ lbs more metal. The total cost was £2.11.7d (casting £1.5s, additional metal at sixteen pence a pound £1.0.8d, carriage both ways 2/-d, hanging and materials 3/9d, beer at the hanging 2d).[9]

Abbot's Hospital Guildford

Maurice Abbot continued to be interested in the hospital until his death in 1678. His knowledge of his family made it possible for him to recommend several former servants of the founder as residents or out-brothers or sisters. One of these was William Harrison, the Archbishop's tailor, admitted in great poverty in March 1660, and given a loan to buy things needed in his room. For many years he made the hospital gowns. Sometimes grants were made to those whom George Abbot had employed, when they had fallen on hard times.

There were also founder's kin who were assisted. The Archbishop's youngest brother John's daughter Sarah married twice. In 1658 Charles Saye, one of her sons by her first husband Robert Saye, was given a grant of £5, as he "had bin taken at Sea", a prisoner. By her second husband, Sarah had a son, George Frisby, who lived in poverty in London. At Maurice Abbot's request he was given financial assistance from 1659, and was admitted as an out-brother in May 1665. He died in 1674. His widow, Frances, became an out-sister in December 1675. She also received gifts of money, including £3 in 1681 "towards the putting out of her Son". She died as an in-sister in 1695. John Parsons, the son of James Parsons, Mayor of Guildford in 1618, 1626 and 1635, became an out-brother in 1669. He claimed kinship with the founder, but the relationship has not been traced. The grants which have been mentioned were often from manufacture funds.

Holland managed the affairs of the foundation in his own way, and without much regard for the provisions of the statutes. They were, however, copied for Archbishop William Juxon. Holland took it to London in 1663, for Archbishop Gilbert Sheldon, who had succeeded Juxon that year.[10] The master kept all the records himself, and paid himself the clerk's fee of £1. There is no mention of the secret reserve, and "dead pay", which should have been added to it, was put into the ordinary income, and treated like money coming in from fines when leases were renewed. For example, when the Charlwood lease was renewed in 1676, the hospital funds received half the fine, £5, and the other half was divided into twenty-one shares of 4/6d for the brothers and sisters, the master receiving two shares, according to the statutes. From 1672 to 1687 Holland employed John Wonham, who was paid to visit the farms and make copies of leases. Wonham spent the last five months of his life as a brother in the hospital, until his death in March 1689.

Merrow farm failed to produce its full rent of £80 for several years, only £75 being received. Contravening statute 21, Holland lent £100 to Peter Bettesworth (probably a relation) and used the £6 interest to make up the shortfall in the Merrow rent. In 1679 the rent of Merrow was reduced to £76, and that of Rumbeams at Ewhurst was increased from £27.10s to £31.10s. This is the only alteration made to the annual revenue from the foundation farms. During these years, timber grown on the farms was used extensively for repairs to buildings, but no proper account of it was kept.

Holland kept up a prolonged resistance to payment of the hearth tax for the rooms of the brothers and sisters. His own lodging had five hearths, and there were five in the public rooms. These were admitted as taxable, but the master claimed that the poor residents'

The Hospital 1633-1864

rooms should be exempt. In 1687 he gave way, and paid arrears of £4 for four and a half years. Thereafter he paid £2.10s until 1689, after which the tax was abolished.

After the great fire of London in 1666, there was nervousness about outbreaks in other towns. Guildford acquired a fire engine, and the hospital contributed £1 towards it in 1671. In the following year a dozen buckets were bought for £3 at the request of the mayor and magistrates. Iron hooks to hang them on cost 4/4d. The garden house was built in 1681-2.

In 1683 William Sancroft, who had succeeded Sheldon as Archbishop of Canterbury in 1678, asked Holland to go to Lambeth to give an account of the hospital statutes, and of its condition. A copy of the charter was made for the Archbishop. There was anxiety caused by the cancelling and renewing of some charters by Charles II and James II, and Sancroft wished to be certain that Abbot's foundation was secure.

In the summer of 1685, chapter 12 of the statutes, which generally forbade strangers to stay in the hospital, but permitted the master "to lodge either his friend, or some other person or persons of qualitie" when "there may be extraordinary concourse unto the Towne", was applied for a notable reason. James Scott, Duke of Monmouth, and illegitimate son of Charles II and Lucy Walter, landed at Lyme Regis on 11 June, intending to drive James II from the throne. Five days later he was deprived of his dukedom of Monmouth, but on 20 June he was proclaimed king at Taunton. His rebellion ended with his defeat at Sedgemoor on 6 July and his capture in a ditch in the New Forest. He asked to be taken to the King, and on the way spent the night of 12 July in the "evidence house" over the hospital gateway.[11] James rejected his nephew's plea for mercy, and Scott was executed on Tower Hill on 15 July. Holland's long mastership ended with his death on 6 July 1691. He was buried at Holy Trinity two days later. The new master, elected on 6 July, was Samuel Shaw, an elderly apothecary, aged about 78, whose younger brother, John, was already one of the hospital's brethren. The Shaw family is found in the registers of St Mary's and Holy Trinity from their beginning until early in the nineteenth century, and several members were apothecaries.

Shaw's years as master were uneventful. From 1691 to 1697 no fuel income was received from West Wantley, and only wood was bought. The farm was part of an estate that was seized by the Crown because a trustee, John Caryll, was suspected of dishonest dealings. It was restored by Act of Parliament. No account was kept of the secret reserve from the time of its return from London until 1695, when its value was recorded as £113.19s. It remained at this level for the rest of Shaw's mastership.[12] Unlike Holland, Shaw employed a clerk, but the master did some of the book-keeping, and it was not systematic. Nonetheless, expenditure was kept within the limits of income, averaging £196.10s a year, and he left a balance in the running stock. Shaw died on 9 August 1702, and was buried at Holy Trinity four days later.

The last brother to be admitted to the hospital by Samuel Shaw was Samuel Barton, a vintner, on 27 May 1699. On the day of Shaw's death, Barton, "one of the bretheren of this Hospitall being a man of good name and fame and otherwise qualifyed... was translated from the brotherhood to the Mastership" – the only time, so far, that this has happened. Barton's years were quiet. Like Shaw he employed a clerk, and also did part of the work himself. He understood accounts, and tried to observe the founder's directions. His average annual expenditure was £197.17.10d, within the income, and he continued to increase the balance in the running stock, which Shaw had built up from nothing, and left £73.14.6d. A typical act was the replacement of the silver money in the secret reserve, 7/6d, with current coins; he sold the obsolete silver. Barton died on 12 October 1709, and on 16th was buried at Holy Trinity.

The morning after Barton's death, Robert Berry was chosen to succeed him. Berry was a timber merchant, and his family had been in Guildford at least since the late sixteenth century. He was a magistrate, and had been churchwarden at St Nicolas' in 1688, and Mayor in 1700. He had been in a position to observe local affairs, and was very critical of Holland's conduct of the hospital. As master he was now able to examine the records, and left notes of his disapproval. At first he reckoned that Holland's neglect of the hospital's interests had cost it "mor then iioo ponds in timber and deed pay". Later he modified this to "A greet deall", and in the meanwhile he had set about increasing the income of the foundation. He kept detailed records - in his own hand for the first seven years, with assistance for preparing the statements of accounts. He also noted incidents in the life of the hospital, and the way that national events affected it.

Although agriculture flourished in the early years of the eighteenth century, the prosperity of its farms brought no benefit to the hospital, which received only the fixed rents negotiated by the founder, who ordered in chapter 28 of the statutes that they must not be varied. The annual income was no longer sufficient to meet expenditure, which rose to £218, and the weekly allowance to the residents two shillings and sixpence, was not enough for them. During his mastership, Berry thought of ways to increase the income, but he took an important step quite soon. In March 1712, with the approval of Archbishop Tenison, Tankerleys farm at Dorking was bought, approximately thirty acres adjoining Mereden farm. The price, £113.13.6d, was found mainly from the sale of timber. The rent was £5.10s, which was to be divided among the brothers and sisters on 29 October.[13] In February 1718 Berry bought four acres at Merrow, with a house, for £160 - a high price, but there was young timber on the land. The rent from this, known as Merrow Small farm, was £6.10s, and this was to be added to the general income of the hospital.

Berry understood that the most important product of the farms was timber. Wood was used for repairs at the hospital, and to farm buildings, and there was also a supply of fuel. He tried to ensure that trees were not cut until they were fully grown, so that the best profit would be made, and he would supply wood from elsewhere when it was needed. Some of the farmers, however, were understandably more interested in their own prosperity than that of the hospital, and did not co-operate. Berry also valued fruit trees, and planted one hundred and twelve large apple trees at the new farm at Merrow. When he became master, Edward Smith of Guildford gave him four walnut trees, three

The Hospital 1633-1864

of which he planted in the courtyard and one in the lower garden. Later on he was able to plant more than two hundred young trees at Merrow, which he had grown from the product of the hospital trees. As well as growing vegetables and flowers in the garden, Berry stocked it with gooseberries, apricots, nectarines, pears, cherries and apples, and there were vines. He made sure that the garden was well watered in 1712 and 1714, when drought caused food prices to rise.

The main improvement Berry made to the fabric of the hospital was beginning the work of reducing the size of the large fireplaces in the residents' rooms, in 1713. As at other times the wooden railings in front of the hospital needed to be repaired. Gates were added to the railings in 1710, and the entrance at that point was paved with marble. When he came to the hospital Berry gave the large Elizabethan table, which remains in the boardroom. He also gave a bedstead, without a canopy, costing thirty-five shillings, with a feather bed and bolster (5/-), to improve the furnishing of the master's lodging.

Rising costs affected the feasts that Abbot had instituted, and for which he allowed ten shillings. Berry's first feast, the founder's birthday, shortly after his election, cost fifteen shillings and twopence. Three years later a peak was reached (19/8^1/$_2$d) and Berry began to plan economy. At Easter 1714 he distributed ten shillings among the brothers and sisters, and after that the birthday feast was the only one to be held, costing as much as one pound four shillings in 1717. On the other occasions there was a distribution of money. A modest two shillings was spent in October 1714 "when the Kinge was crowned to be merry with the Brethren".

The approach to Christmas 1713 was marred by the theft of money from the poor-box in the chapel. The whole community suspected Thomas Terry, a brother who was the key-keeper. His lock was found undone, while the other was broken. Terry was called before a formidable tribunal - the master, the vice-master Andrew Powell, the Mayor, Joseph Benbrick, the Rector of Holy Trinity, Michael Woodward, and the head master, Samuel Pigott. He was warned "to live a quiett life", or to be expelled.

Earlier in 1713, three shillings and eightpence was spent on candles, for the celebrations on 4 May for the proclamation of the treaty of Utrecht, ending the eleven years of war with France. Candles were also bought in 1714 when George I was proclaimed, and when he arrived in London, for his coronation, and in 1715, when there was a thanksgiving day "for all gods Blessens in given us A protestant Kinge". The candles were burnt in the windows, to save them from being broken by revellers in the street. The use seems to have worked.

In 1714 trouble was caused by the Mayor, John Smallpeice, who insisted on placing his own brother, Thomas, in the hospital, though he was under age and known to be a trouble-maker. Berry gave way, but recorded his protest in the ledger. In 1718 it was discovered that Thomas was brewing gin in one of the main rooms in the hospital, and spoiling the ceiling. Berry expelled him, but the Mayor, John Goodyer, and the Rector of Holy

Trinity, Edward Vernon, prevailed on Berry to keep him. Thomas continued to live riotously, rarely attending church or chapel, and was still a brother when Berry died.

Berry's health began to fail in 1716, and he took steps to help his successor to continue to improve the stability of the foundation. He bought a new book, Ledger II, and entered copies of the leases of the hospital farms. He strongly recommended that leases should not be long, and that the tenants should not be allowed to assign them to others. It should be ensured that the hospital's rights in the farms should be secured, especially in the use of timber. If economy was observed, for example by having new gowns only every four years, it should be possible to increase the weekly distribution to three shillings, or even 3/6d.

Berry died in December 1719, most probably on 17th. He is remembered as one of the best masters of the hospital, and shewed that a revision of Abbot's arrangements was necessary for the well-being of the community.

The next master was Thomas Sands, a saddler, whose family is found in local registers since 1628. There is no record of his election, but he began his accounting on 17 December. Sands, who was a widower, caused comments by wearing his municipal gown, instead of the master's. He was not a businessman, and the hospital accounts were kept incompletely and inaccurately - worse than at any other time. In 1721 he completed Berry's scheme of reducing the size of the fireplaces, to save fuel. Sands also improved the staircase in the northern range, which was found to be too steep. As built it rose in one flight to a gallery on the north wall. As reconstructed in 1721, it rose more gently to a half-landing, and then returned to a gallery on the south wall, as it still does.

The most important event of Sands's mastership was the Archbishop's visitation. William Wake became Archbishop in 1716, and in 1721 sent John Bettesworth, Official Principal of the Court of Arches, to conduct the visitation as his commissary. This was not part of a provincial visitation, and it is not known why Wake decided to take this action. The enquiry discovered no corruption, but a sad level of slackness, and this was revealed in the orders and injunctions of 25 November 1721, which the master was to read to the brothers and sisters, called to the chapel for the purpose.

1. There had been irregularities when a new master was chosen. In the future, before an election, the Rector of Holy Trinity – or in his absence the Rector of St Nicolas', was to read, audibly and distinctly, the third chapter of the hospital statutes, and also the relevant clause in the sixth statute of 31 Queen Elizabeth, which declared void any election of this kind if it was found that money had been paid to secure it. It was not suggested that this offence had been committed

2. Not all the residents had taken the prescribed oaths, and were to do so within three weeks.

3. No-one was to be admitted below the age of sixty. John Stevens, one of the brothers, who had been admitted in 1720, was found to be under age, and order was given to "amove" him.[14]

4. Good discipline and behaviour were to be maintained. The troublesome Thomas Smallpeice was once again expelled.

5. The master was to wear his hospital gown, for which he received an allowance, and not his councillor's gown

6. The regulations in the statutes for the payment of rents to the hospital had not been observed, and this was to be corrected. All money was to be received in the hospital itself, and the audit was to made as the statutes required. The rents from the newly acquired properties were to be distributed to the master and residents. This frustrated Berry's intention that the income from Merrow small farm should increase the hospital income.

7. Greater care was to be taken in the management of timber on the hospital estates; no trees were to be felled without the Archbishop's consent. It was discovered that £76.2.4½d was owed to Sands, and that the secret reserve was short by £11. Timber due to be cut would be sufficient to make up these sums.

8. On market days some people had been permitted to put loads of corn in the shelter of the entrance gateway. The master was to forbid this.

9. The master had been claiming the garden as his own. It was maintained at the common expense, so it belonged to the whole community. However, to secure fairness, the master was to keep the key, and be asked for it when brothers and sisters wanted to get root vegetables or greens. Fruit was to be gathered and taken to the common hall, to be distributed among the residents.

10. The requirements of chapter 7 of the statutes regarding chapel and church attendance, and receiving Holy Communion, were to be observed, and all should live consistently with this: "in the mean time to make yo'selves worthy Communicants thereof by Denying Ungodliness and worldly Lusts, and living Soberly Righteously and Godly in this present World".

These orders and injunctions were an attempt to restore life in the hospital to the standards set by the founder; only the rules for the garden were new. Heed was not taken of Berry's advice, and no thought was given to augmenting the income to match the rise in the cost of living.

A link with the past came to an end on 8 October 1723, when Elizabeth Clarke, one of the sisters died. She was the last member of the hospital community "whome was related to the Bishup", and it was recorded in the ledger. She had been admitted as an in-sister in 1708, having had an annual allowance of five or six shillings since 1699. Sands died on 17 June 1729, and was buried at Holy Trinity.

Thomas Sands died at 3 o'clock in the morning, and between ten and eleven the same morning Ephraim Wood was chosen to succeed him. Although this was the first election since the Archbishop's visitation, the formalities do not seem to have been observed;

neither the death nor the admission was recorded in the ledger, and neither rector was present when Wood was elected. Wood was a barber and peruke-maker. He kept limited records, and there is no mention at all of timber, or of the appointment of vice-master or nurses. Sometimes he gave precise details, however. For the Christmas dinner of 1730, for example, 15/2d was spent (meat 8/2d, bread 2/-d, flour, raisins, sugar, currants, eggs, salt, butter and milk 5/-d). Admonitions for abuse and drunkenness were recorded as usual, as when Samuel Trasey had to be carried home from St Catherine's fair on 15 October 1731. Wood died on 2 May 1734.

The new master, chosen on 3 May, was Henry Stoughton, described as a chapman. The Rector of Holy Trinity, William Bannaster, was present in the hospital that day. Stoughton acted as his own clerk, and kept his records methodically if not neatly. He had an increase in disciplinary problems, especially drunkenness and quarrelling, among both the men and the women, and cases are recorded in painful detail in ledger II. These are examples. In 1737, Daniel Wicks abused the master roundly, "and tould the Master he Could talk a Spider to an Ox and an Ox to a Spider and talk a Mans Coat of from his back... The Master told Wicks he should not frequent Alehouses so often, Wicks's answer was, then you must stand at the Door... And Wick told the Master, do you take Care of Yourself and other reprochfull Languaigd." In 1739, Elizabeth Pell was fined 2/6d four times within a month for abusing another sister. "On Sunday June the 12: 1743 Hugh Kettle Vice Master, Tho: Roberts Henry Larkins all a Drinking of Gin, till Eleven a Clock at night. Kettle and Roberts going to their Roomes Roberts fell Down Kettle told him he could not help him upp, so Roberts crawled on his hands & knees to Kettles Roome and Lay on the floor all Night, as he Confesses himself: but Kettle said he came in to Light his pipe and fell down in a fett etc."

In 1740 considerable excitement was provided by events on the other side of the High Street. Holy Trinity Church had become increasingly dilapidated, and it was decided to close it for repairs. The last service was held on Saturday 19 April. On the following Wednesday, 23 April, while the bells were being lowered, the steeple fell through the roof of the nave. Remarkably no-one was injured, even though the street was crowded at the time. There was a surprising lack of haste in replacing the church. The ruins were not demolished until 1749, and another fourteen years elapsed before the new building was first used, on 18 September 1763. The tomb of Archbishop Abbot was not damaged in the disaster. It was taken down and stored in the hospital until it could be re-erected in the new church. It is traditionally thought that the seats in the hospital chapel may be from the old Holy Trinity Church, rescued and used to replace less comfortable, and probably backless, benches provided by the founder.

In 1742 a Mr Goodyer was paid £7.11.8d for a clock, and this was set up in the north range. It is probable that the mechanism was second hand.[15] In preparation, a turret was made on the roof, costing £2.15s, and the bell was moved there from the north-east turret of the gate house, so that the hours could be struck.

The Hospital 1633-1864

Henry Stoughton died early in the morning on 27 July 1744. A few hours later Hugh Moth, a barge master, was chosen, in the presence of the Rector of Holy Trinity. The five years of this mastership were uneventful. Moth acted as his own clerk, and like his predecessor was methodical but not tidy. He ignored the injunctions of Archbishop Wake, who had died in 1737, with respect to the income from Merrow small farm. Instead of dividing it among the master and residents, he added it to the general hospital income – as Berry intended when he bought the farm. This irregularity continued until George White became master. Moth died on 18 June 1749, and was buried at St Mary's the same day, a Sunday, which also saw the election of his successor, William Goodyer.

Goodyer, a cooper, was master for longer than any of his predecessors, except only Holland, over thirty years. He employed William Gumm as clerk, and was himself a good manager, and like Moth before him, ran the hospital economically. Timber on the farms was maturing, and was cut both for sale and for hospital repairs. In 1756 much was brought in from Merrow for use, and a sawpit was dug in the garden, at a cost of 2/6d. A "Cloath and Lacing for the Desk board in the Chappell" was bought for three shillings - one of the few liturgical ornaments available for decoration in those times.

The average yearly expenditure under Goodyer was £199, and the balance of savings grew, reaching £252.1.9³/₄d by November 1759. On 11 April 1760 bank stock was purchased – £200, costing £221.10s, with the broker's fee of five shillings added. This produced a half-yearly income of £4.10s, which was divided among the community.

Goodyer died on 3 October 1762, and on the same day the second clerical master was elected, Cornelius Jeale, of St John's College Oxford, and, like Holland, a Gloucestershire man. Jeale was well known in Guildford as head master of the Grammar School from 1733 to 1756. He became Rector of Wisley and perpetual curate of Pyrford on 30 July 1736, and held those parishes until his death, even though he lived in Guildford, and acted as curate at St Nicolas' from about 1754.[16] He did not take the oath as master when he was elected because he was ill. On the following day he climbed to the treasury to inspect the silver and the old gold. By now the secret reserve had become a collection of obsolete coins, which were weighed for their value as bullion - less than half the face value. Twenty-five days later Jeale died, on 29 October, and was buried at Holy Trinity on 3 November.

On the day that Cornelius Jeale died, a cooper, Michael Wallis was elected by the Mayor, Laurence Ledger, the vice-master, John Warwick, and the senior brothers, Samuel Goodwin and George Flint. The rectors, Charles Burdet of Holy Trinity and Thomas Lowe of St Nicolas', were not present, but the election was witnessed by Peter Flutter, John Martyr and the clerk William Gumm. In the little less than six and a half years that Wallis was master, much was done to improve the financial well-being of the charity and its management. He was helped by the advice of several leading townsmen, Henry and Peter Flutter and Thomas Jackman, all of whom served as Mayor, and the town clerk John Martyr. The books were kept mainly by William Gumm, who was succeeded as clerk on his death early in 1763 by his son George.

Abbot's Hospital Guildford

A higher income was needed to improve the lot of the residents, who could not pay their way with their slender allowance. Some of the men went out to work, as allowed by the statutes, and some of the sisters worked as nurses. Early in 1764, Wallis persuaded the brethren that the silver bowls and salts, which were not used at feasts, and the gold coins were "dead stock", and that they should be sold to provide fruitful stock. The silver, apart from four spoons,[17] was bought by John Murray for £36.11.1d (at 5/2d an ounce), Martyr acting as the agent. The gold coins were sold for £39.9.9d. With these two sums and £38.9.2d from hospital funds, was bought bank stock - £100 for £114.7.6d, with a broker's fee of half a crown. In 1765 £300 more bank stock was bought for £383.12.6d. The money for this was raised by the sale of timber, for £711.10s, the balance being put into the general fund. In 1763 there is the first mention of fire insurance, with the Sun Fire Office. The first payment was £1.7.6d, on policy 423632.[18]

In January 1764 the founder's tomb was reassembled in the new Holy Trinity Church, at the cost of £3.10.9d, which included 2/6d for beer for the workmen.[19]

Care for the hospital property was shewn in 1764. On 9 June, the master and brethren unanimously decided to bring an action against John Lingfield of Coolhurst near Horsham for trespassing on Highlands farm, and felling and removing two oak trees. John Martyr acted for the hospital when the case was heard at Lewes Castle in August 1765. The verdict was given for the hospital. Lingfield paid £53 to Martyr; the tenant, Mr Hurst, paid £13.6.8d, and the hospital £30.13.6d. Martyr's bill of costs exceeded £93.

Merrow farm was held on a twenty-one year lease by John Searle, and it was to expire at Michaelmas 1765. Searle was responsible for repairs, but it was accepted that the house was too large and ruinous for this to be insisted on. The cost of repairs was estimated at £285.12.9d excluding timber, which would be taken from the farm. The Archbishop of Canterbury, Thomas Secker, was asked to approve of the scheme for repairing the house. He asked the Rector of Holy Trinity, Burdet, for a report. Burdet took advice, and recommended that the rent should be increased to not less than £100 in the new lease, that a new house should be bought, and that the materials from the old house should be used for repairing farm buildings. Secker replied to Burdet on 23 March 1765, giving his opinion, that Searle should pay £68 in lieu of repairs, that the rent should be increased, that a fine of £100 should be paid for the new lease, and that a new house might be provided. Money was raised by the sale of timber, £674.10s, and a new farmhouse was built for £400. Searle was fortunate. He had the benefit of a new house, he paid a fine of only £20, and he continued to pay the same rent, £76, with £5.19s for the small farm; and he did not pay the £68 in place of repairs. Some of the panelling from the old farmhouse was used in the new, and some was brought to the hospital, possibly for the master's bedroom.

In 1768 the £600 bank stock was sold for £998.6s, securing a profit of £279.16s. Woolpits farm at Ewhurst, rather more than 93 acres, was purchased for £969.3s. The balance of the sale price of the bank stock, £29.3s, was put into the general fund. The first half year's rent from Woolpits farm was £13.5s, of which £1.3.7½d was tax.

The Hospital 1633-1864

Wallis's attention to detail brought twenty-three shillings to the hospital in 1763. A neighbour, Mr Mabanke, paid sixpence a year for encroachment - an accumulation of forty-six years, and was given permission to retain the building that he had put up against the west wall of the hospital. In 1766 the hospital received a legacy under the will of Henry Flutter, £100 "towards the augmentation of that charity".

By good management, Wallis brought about a marked improvement in the hospital's affairs, even though the rents were still at the rate that Abbot left them, and the fines on leases were little increased. His average expenditure was £195, and he was able to add six and a half pence to the weekly distribution of 2/6d.

Wallis's active mastership ended with his death on 12 March 1769. On the same day George Lovedale White was elected. Like Wallis he was a cooper, and had been baptized at Holy Trinity on 1 January 1702. George Gumm continued to keep the cash account. No admonitions or forfeits were recorded, and the keeping of the ledger was allowed to lapse. The accounts were signed by the brethren on 9 November 1772, but there was no further audit while White was master. The reason noted was that the people responsible were dead, or "in too indigent circumstances to admit the hope of any good being likely to arise from an expensive investigation of this neglect". Entries in the ledger stopped on 2 September 1773. It may be that White wished to conceal an irregular transaction. On 19 May 1770, James Woolley, a bricklayer, entered into a bond with the master for £200, as was discovered after White's death. This was contravening chapter 21 of the statutes.

Another farm was bought - Salthurst, adjoining Woolpits at Ewhurst. The land, sixteen and a half acres, was bought from J. Martyn for £220, advance payment of £73.2.11d in 1771 and the balance of £146.17.1d in 1772. Peter Flutter made a gift of £100 to the hospital some time before his death on 6 January 1771. This was used for this purchase, and £120 was raised by the sale of timber from Highlands farm. In 1772, the foundation farms produced £200, following the recent rearrangements. The private farms, as those purchased after the foundation were called, produced £41.13.11d (Merrow small farm £5.19s, Tanklings £5.10s, Woolpits £23.3.5d, Salthurst £7.1.6d) with the tax deducted.

The Reverend William Cole came to Guildford on one of his antiquarian journeys in 1774, and visited the hospital. He considered that the room over the hall was "of no use, but to have Balls in, now & then for the Town". He found that prayers in the chapel were conducted by a layman "in a blew Coat & Brass Buttons", presumably the master, who "said of his own free Motion [that he] 'would not suffer any Clergymn to be concerned in this Service'. Was not this taking the lowest of the People, and making them Priests of the Lord?"[20]

White died on 18 May 1778, and was buried at Holy Trinity three days later. On 18 May, the Reverend Edmund Brewer was elected. Brewer, who came from Penrith in Cumberland, was a graduate of Queen's College Oxford, and was Rector of Puttenham from 1752 to 1776. He lived in Guildford, in St Nicolas' parish, and acted as curate there from about 1760.

Brewer employed as clerk Anne Webster. On 5 January 1779 she was married at Pirbright parish Church to the Reverend Thomas Townsend, the Rector, who was also curate at Worplesdon. They appear to have lived at the hospital, and Townsend succeeded his wife as clerk. A daughter was born to them in the hospital on 8 January 1780, but the pleasurable interest that this gave to the brothers and sisters was shortlived, for the mother died twelve days later. Townsend officiated at Pirbright until April 1797, and is said to have committed suicide soon after that.

A fire broke out in the brewhouse, probably in May 1779, but the cost of the repairs cannot be extracted from the sums spent on maintenance in the first months of Brewer's mastership. Thomas Attfield received 10/8d for smiths's work; James Clarke for bricklaying and tiling, £2.8.6d; Joseph Jennings £27.10.9¼d for glazier's work, including £7.4.6¾d arrears from White's time; John Upton £21.3.7½d for bricklaying and plastering, and "for putting up the Copper again which was taken down to stop the fire"; Thomas Upton £7.11.5d for carpenter's work - a total of £59.4.11¾d. It was noted that on receiving payment, John Upton put three pence into the poor box, whereas Jennings gave 7/6d. During the whole of his time as master, Brewer spent £148.17.6d on repairs, which were paid by the sale of timber from Burstow (£80) and Charlwood (£115). A survey of the farms was made on 31 August 1779 and the following day by Thomas Upton, with the vice-master and clerk. The survey cost £1.11.6d (presumably for food, drink and lodging) and horses were hired from Attfield for £2.5s, including duty 3s. At Rumbeams and Highlands the buildings were found to be in poor repair. During the survey they proposed to sell timber worth £340, and this paid for repairs to the hospital and farms.

Life in the hospital at this time was not very eventful, and despite the efforts to increase the income, the amount paid to the brothers and sisters was still meagre, and prices continued to rise. A welcome gift came with a legacy of £50 from Dr James Price of Stoke, to be divided among the twenty residents. Brewer tried to recover the £200 from James Woolley by persuading him to take up the bond. £50 was received in January 1780, and interest a few times, but then it was apparently forgotten. Some of the brethren fell on evil days. William Cox died in the workhouse on 5 February 1780. He had been there for a fortnight, and was allowed 2/6d a week. His body was returned to the hospital for burial at the parish's expense. A year later "Joseph Ford being unhappily afflicted with a Bodily Infirmity which renders him a Nuisance to this Society" was dismissed, but was to remain an out-brother.

Brewer died on 22 February 1784, and was buried at Holy Trinity five days later. The next master was Edward Brinkwell, who was elected on 23 February. He was a plumber, and had been Mayor of Guildford in 1772 and 1782. The routine of inspecting the chest was still carried out by new masters, even after the sale of the gold coins and most of the silver in 1764. Brinkwell found £155.17s, in notes and coins, and also Woolley's bond, now for £150.

The Hospital 1633-1864

Extra income, badly needed by the hospital, was provided by one of its major benefactors, Alderman Thomas Jackman. He had been Mayor in 1764, 1774 and 1783, and was familiar with the foundation's difficulties. His augmentation was achieved in two stages. In 1779, Jackman bought some land at Albury, from John and Sarah Smither of Bramley, for £600. There was a charge on this sum, which Smither and his wife, or their heirs, were to pay until the land was redeemed. On 25 March 1785, Jackman, in consideration of a payment by the hospital of ten shillings, made over his interest in the £600 and the land. The income was to give an extra sixpence each week to the brothers and sisters, an annual sum of ten shillings to the clerk, and £1 for a feast every year on 11 April. Newcomers were not eligible for the first quarter of a year, and the 6/6d saved was to be added to the April feast sum. Any balance was to be given to the master.

The second stage was of a different kind. Jackman persuaded the Mayor and the magistrates to apply to the Court of Chancery for a variation of the manufacture's financial rules.[21] It was claimed that the distribution to poor tradesmen encouraged idleness, in the expectation of gifts. An order in chancery of 14 December 1785 reduced the amount for distribution to £50; the remaining £50 was diverted to the hospital, with effect from the beginning of 1786. Four additional sisters were to be received, bringing the number of women to twelve, equal to the men. Rooms for them were found by using the porter's lodge, by reclaiming and dividing a room by the master's lodging, which had been used as additional accommodation by masters, and by creating a room by the stairs from the old kitchen. The doors of these rooms were marked "Mr J". These four sisters were to receive 3/4d every week, a total of £34.13.4d a year. The rest was apportioned - £3 for new gowns in alternate years (£1.10s each), £1.6.8d for fuel (6/8d each), gaudy day dinners 16s, £1 (5/-each) on the Founder's birthday, fuel for the common hall 13/4d. The master was to receive £8.10.8d as rent, or compensation, for the rooms that he had lost. Jackman requested that any of his family, if poor and otherwise qualified, should be admitted to the hospital. The Jackman sisters received less than those of the original foundation, as they were not eligible for a share in occasional income, under the statutes. For this reason, the practice was adopted that all new sisters were at first elected to the new foundation, and then transferred to the old when vacancies allowed.

In 1786 John Smither took up the bond, and the hospital received the £600. This money was not included in the hospital account, but until 1809 was in the hands of the town clerk. £874.6.4d old South Sea annuities were purchased, producing £26.4.4d. The hospital added sufficient to bring the annual income up to £30. In 1789 £300 new South Sea annuities were bought for £225, to increase Jackman's augmentation.

Thomas Jackman died in October 1788. His generosity increased the income of the hospital, and made it possible for there to be a permanent fund of bank stock. The enlarging of the community widened the benefit to the poor of the town. His portrait, painted in 1786 by John Russell, the Guildford artist, now hangs in the boardroom.

The chapel and its services are not mentioned in the records of the hospital under Brinkwell, but the comfort of the worshippers was considered when a padded cushion,

Abbot's Hospital Guildford

or squab, was bought for their pew in Holy Trinity church for six shillings. The hospital shared in the national rejoicing by lighting candles on 16 March 1789, to celebrate the recovery of King George III from his second bout of madness (if such it was), and therefore the end of the short regency of his son George, the Prince of Wales.

Brinkwell died on 30 January 1792. The accounts had been kept up to November 1791, but there was a discrepancy of £200, which the master's executors made good.

On 30 January Richard Elkins, a chapman, was chosen as master, at the age of 58. The seventeen years that followed shewed an improvement in the hospital's finances, partly because of the master's personal generosity. Following the example of Thomas Jackman, Elkins increased the investment in consolidated annuities. In 1804 he noted that he considered that it was better to add to the capital, and so increase the income for the weekly distribution, than to give out the proceeds of fines on lease renewals. By that year he was able to add one shilling to the weekly payments. By the end of 1805 he had income for another sixpence, and he hoped for another similar increase "should the Supreme Being be pleased to preserve my Life so long". Between 1796 and 1.805 stock with a face value of £2160 was bought for £1619.15.2d.[22] Most of the money to pay for this came from the sale of timber, but fines on leases also produced part of it. Further stock was acquired through the benefaction of Jane More Molyneux of Loseley, who left £2000 to the hospital when she died in 1802. This money was held in the name of the Mayor and the Approved Men, and was for the benefit of all the residents. Income that was kept out of the hospital's official accounts could be used for the Jackman sisters as well as those of Abbot's foundation, and helped to raise them to equality. In 1808 a total of £5460 bank stock was held, producing an income of £185.8s.

The master's own contribution came from his declining to receive the allowance for the loss of the rooms now occupied by the Jackman sisters. He made a note of this on 7 April 1797, and also made over the accumulation for the years since he had taken office, £42.15.4d. He hoped that future masters would do the same, but he could not commit them to that. At the end of his mastership, his voluntary augmentation had amounted to £145.1.4d. Part of this was used to buy cloth for the gowns of the Jackman sisters, when the foundation brothers and sisters refused to allow endowment income to be used for them.

The chapel received modest improvements. In 1795 the reading desk was given a cloth with a fringe (18/-) and four hassocks were bought (5/-). In 1796 a brass sconce was bought (1/6d) and a brass candle-stick in 1800 (1/-).

In 1807 a longstanding dispute with the parishioners of Merrow was resolved - the repair of part of the fence of the churchyard, which hospital land adjoined. Elkins called in an eminent lawyer to adjudicate, Michael Nolan, a special pleader on the home circuit and the Surrey sessions. Nolan gave his opinion on 23 August, that the master and brethren were responsible for repairing the fence and keeping it in repair. This was done at a cost of £15.15s. Legal fees were £12.8.6d.

The Hospital 1633-1864

Illuminations with candles became popular, and in 1797 sockets were fixed, costing 4/2d, in readiness to celebrate the battle of Camperdown. The candles were bought for 19/4d. Further illuminations followed in 1798, for the battle of the Nile (10/11d), in 1802, for the peace of Amiens (£1.5.8½d), and in 1805, for the battle of Trafalgar (6/6d).

Only at the beginning and the end of his mastership did Elkins have serious disciplinary problems. In 1793, on two successive days, Henry Potter and Henry Brookes were expelled, with drunkenness as the main reason. In September 1808 another brother was sent out for the same cause. Elkins resigned on 31 January 1809, the first master to do so. He died soon afterwards, on 29 March, and was buried at Holy Trinity on 5 April.

The next master, chosen on 31 January, was Samuel Russell, a member of a well known Guildford family. The Russells are first found in Guildford in 1509. Samuel's grandfather John was a bookseller in the High Street, and was Mayor in 1723. His son, the second John, succeeded in the business, and added printing to its activities. He was Mayor four times. His son John was the artist, mentioned above, and his second son, Samuel, born in 1746, was taken into partnership. Samuel was Mayor in 1805.

Shortly after Russell became master, the hospital received a gift of five paintings from the first Earl of Onslow, the entombment of Christ and portraits of leaders of reformation thought, John Wycliffe, Sebastian Munster, John Foxe and John Calvin.[23] During Russell's years the hospital's bank stock was re-invested. In 1814 £3160 was sold for £2619.4.6d (with commission deducted), and with this £2695.13.1d 5% new navy stock was bought. In the same year and the next, £671.17.8d cash from the hospital fund was used to buy a further £704.6.11d stock, bringing the total to £3400, which produced an annual income of £170. After 1822 this investment was transferred to £3570 4% new navy stock, producing £142.16s, and it stood at that rate at Russell's death.

Repairs began straight away under Russell. In fifteen years £1581.10.6 ¾d was spent on the hospital, as well as £8 on the Founder's tomb.[24] This was mostly raised by the sale of timber (£1045. 19.8½d). Half the fine on the Highlands lease added £440, and the balance of £103.10.10¼d came from general income. Some of the timber that was felled was brought to the hospital for use. The panelling in the presence chamber was repaired at this time. A noticeable alteration was the replacement of the 1741 bell turret with the Gothic structure shewn in Alexander Munro's drawings.

There were illuminations twice while Russell was master. On 19 July 1814 £2.11s was spent when the allied sovereigns, the Emperor Alexander of Russia and Frederick William of Prussia passed through Guildford on their way to Portsmouth. In November 1820 £1.3.4½d was spent "for the Queen's Aquittal" - when George IV's attempt to divorce Queen Caroline failed when the Earl of Liverpool's government decided not to take the bill to the House of Commons. A domestic celebration was held in 1819 for the second centenary of the laying of the stone in 1619. The Easter dinner was held on 8 April, costing £4.12.9½d, but on 24 May the large sum of £22 was spent on a dinner and wine.

Abbot's Hospital Guildford

The rooms of the residents were in some cases improved at their own expense. Some of them had put stoves into the open fireplaces, and some had acquired cupboards. At the very end of Russell's mastership the first gas bill was paid for the hospital, £1.2.6d. Gas became available in Guildford in 1824, and the town was first lit on 4 May. Russell died on 8 May 1824, and was buried at Holy Trinity on 14 May.

Samuel Robinson was chosen to be the next master on the day that Russell died. He was seventy years old, and was the proprietor of the Guildford Arms, an inn just downhill from the Guildhall. The next year, 1825, produced a good income for the hospital. Timber was sold from several farms, and brought in £1170.9s. The renewal of leases at Merrow and Highlands produced fines of £1795, half of which was for general purposes. Bank stock was bought for £1000 in 1826. Much larger fines could now be levied because of agricultural prosperity. In 1825 the carved arms of James I were placed over the main entrance. The mason was paid £47.5s.

Through the years there were frequent references to the fence in front of the hospital. It was decided to replace it with the stone balustrade that is still there. The design was based on that of the old fence, and one object was to give greater protection from the riots that took place in the High Street at election times and on 11 November. The stonework was completed in 1830, the gas lamp was added in 1831, costing £1.3.2d, and the ironwork at the entrance in 1832, for £14.15.10½d. The total cost was £244.17.6d (including £5.5.8d for beer for the workmen) and £109.14s of this was raised by subscriptions.

Life in the hospital was changing. By the time of Robinson's death in 1833, all the rooms had stoves. As they were more cosy, the residents used the common rooms less frequently. The stairs down to the cellars were blocked off, and little sculleries were created in the spaces made there. The statutory feasts were given up from 1828, and a distribution of money was made instead, of one shilling, but two shillings to the Jackman sisters. The feel of community was diminished, only being kept alive by the chapel services and by the maintenance of discipline.

Robinson died on 1 May 1833, and was buried ay Holy Trinity a week later. The next master was Jesse Boxall, chosen on 1 May, aged seventy-one. His wife had died earlier in the year.

Drunkenness was quite often dealt with in these years, and Robinson had been supported by Henry Parr Beloe, who had been Rector of Holy Trinity since 1824. In 1836 Beloe told James Ansell at his third admonition, that if he offended again "it would not only be attended by immediate expulsion, but would place his soul in peril of the punishment of eternal misery". Beloe died in May 1838. Ansell was fined for drunkenness the following month, losing one month's allowances. He proved incorrigible, and in July was discharged for this "and other unproper conduct". The other side of corporate life was made more comfortable, for by 1837 a coke stove had been put into the chapel.

The Hospital 1633-1864

The finances of the hospital had become more complicated, as additional sources of income had been secured. There was no hint of corruption, and the aim of improving the payments to the brothers and sisters was praiseworthy. Nonetheless, a clear distinction was not made between hospital income and brotherhood income. Bank stock was hospital property, but its dividends were used to add to the payments to the brotherhood. Repairs to farm buildings should have been borne by the tenants, but often the hospital paid, and that reduced the profit for general expenses. On the other hand, income was raised when timber was sold. The Jackman sisters were still at the disadvantage of not sharing in the distribution from fines on leases, but some new income was equally for their benefit. Mrs Iredell left £200 to the hospital, which was received in 1843. It was to be invested, to produce 1s.1d annually for each brother and sister. When interest rates fell, the hospital made up the difference, so that the income of the residents was not reduced.

Boxall died on 18 February 1846, and was buried at St Mary's. In accordance with custom, following chapter 3 of the statutes, the new master was chosen on the day of Boxall's death; but the future would be different from the past. The age of reform had begun.

---

1. The inventory is printed in Palmer 1917 pp 38f, with detailed notes on the contents, and information about what happened to them in future years, pp 39-53.

2. This great vessel seems to have been replaced in 1809 by the large "Pottage Pot" that is now used for flowers in the garden (£1.6.6d, allowing for old metal).

3. All that remains of this silver is three of the spoons, with another of similar pattern. The rest was sold a century later. Mr Stephen Clarke of Christies, in a letter of 30 December 1986, recorded the slip-top spoons:

    1. James Cluatt, London 1606 or 1608
    2. William Scarborough, London 1624
    3. probably John Freake, London 1624
    4. probably Adam King, London mark indistinct (but previously noted as 1669)

4. For the course of the war in Surrey, see Maldon 1905 pp 228-251.

5. A rough wooden box in the boardroom, covered with skin, is traditionally said to be that which was made for this emergency.

6. The Book of Common Prayer was banned by an ordinance of Parliament on 3 January 1645, the day that the bill of attainder of William Laud was passed by the House of Lords, and a week before his execution.

7. See chapter 3 above p 34.

8. The corn and fulling mills had been given to trustees in 1643 by Henry Smith, for the benefit of Guildford's poor.

Abbot's Hospital Guildford

9. The bell has an inscription – "WE.1662". William Eldridge, who died in 1716, was the last known member of a family of bellfounders first heard of at Wokingham in 1565.
10. Holland's copy has not survived, but the original Lambeth copy had not, after all, been lost in the damage done to the palace in 1640.
11. James Scott, whom Charles II acknowledged as his son, was created Duke of Monmouth and Earl of Doncaster on 14 February 1663, and Duke of Buccleuch and Earl of Dalkeith in the Scottish peerage on 20 April 1663.
12. The store of money was made up of 43 old gold coins, valued by weight at £46.9s; 60 guineas worth 22/- each and one guinea worth 22/6d; some silver coins worth 7/6d. Guineas were first coined in 1663, and it is probable that these were paid in by Holland's executors.
13. This was known at first as the "birthday gift" and later as the "fairday gift", and its origin was not remembered.
14. He was readmitted by Sands when he was old enough.
15. Mr G.G. Stevens, the Guildford horologist, who maintained and repaired the clock for many years from 1956, considered that it could have been made at any time between 1400 and 1600, and that it had been altered, probably when it was installed. No illustration of this first bell turret is known.
16. For comments on incumbents who served also as curates, see Taylor 1980 pp 9f.
17. See note 3, above.
18. In 1793 a new policy (611266) for £600 was taken out, the premium being twelve shillings.
19. When the church was enlarged in 1888, the tomb was moved to its present position. Palmer noted that some of the marble had been put back upside down in 1764. This was corrected in 1888.
20. Cole had in mind the sin of Jeroboam, 1 Kings 12,31 and 13,33.
21. See chapter 3.
22. The record of the purchase of bank stock:

date	face value	cost (excluding fees & commission)	source of money
2/8/1796	£500	£191. 15. 0d	timber at Highlands, Mereden & Tanklings; half fine for Charlwood
27/2/1798	£150	£90. 18. 9d	timber at Tanklings & Meriden; share of annuities surrendered by master
27/4/1802	£50	£46. 0. 0d	timber from Rumbeams;
8/7/1802	£100	£96. 7. 6d	half fine
5/7/1803	£100	£65. 5. 0d	from Burstow
7/7/1803	£50	£34. 6. 3d	timber from Tanklings
11/8/1803	£50	£34. 7. 6d	& Mereden
31/5/1804	£100	£71. 15. 0d	timber from Highlands,

26/6/1804	£150	£108. 15. 0d	Charlwood,
14/7/1804	£250	£186. 0. 0d	Burstow & Merrow; half fine for Burstow
27/4/1805	£536.17.6d	£399. 6. 0d	half fine for Merrow
13/6/1805	£123. 2.6d	£ 92. 19. 2d	timber from Mereden

23 The pictures were brought from the Friary, which had been owned by the Onslow family since 1736. The gift also included the bloodstained chair in which an earlier owner of the Friary, Daniel Colwall, treasurer of the Royal Society, had shot himself in 1690. Lord Onslow died in 1814, and the Friary, which had been used as a barracks since 1794, was demolished by his son, the second earl, in 1818.

24. In August 1817 the tomb was also cleaned with vinegar, at a cost of 4/2d.

Abbot's Hospital Guildford

FIVE
THE REFORMED COMMUNITY

Andrew Hooke was elected to follow Boxall on 18 February 1846. He was a land surveyor, who had worked on the surveys of Nightingale Road and Boxgrove Road. Aged about seventy-four, he had been a widower since 1801. For many years he was parish clerk of Holy Trinity. His church interests were shewn by modest improvements to the chapel, a cushion and stool in the pulpit and two stools and two mats in the master's pew in 1846, a hole in the ceiling stopped and a ventilator fixed in 1847, a purple cloth for the reading desk, four kneeling stools and two deal stools covered with Dutch carpet in 1848, cleaning, repairing and varnishing the stalls and pews in 1852, and three cocoa mats in 1853. There were regular repairs to the mullions and glass of the chapel windows. However, the records of Hooke's time reveal anxiety about the finances of the hospital, at a time when public interest had been roused and when scandal was eagerly exposed.

In 1812 an Act of Parliament had been passed "to provide a summary remedy in cases of abuses of Trusts created for Charitable Purposes". Desire to promote the common good mingled with spirited curiosity brought all kinds of charitable bodies and institutions under scrutiny, and in many cases abuses were found. The lively but not accurate *The Black Book* of 1820 and its successors, the two issues of *The Extraordinary Black Book* in 1831 and 1832 fired imaginations. The most notorious case was that of St Cross Hospital at Winchester, and its master Francis North, who succeeded to the earldom of Guilford in 1827.[1] This began to occupy the newspapers in 1843.

A survey, *The Charities in the County of Surrey* was published in 1839, with a section on Guildford.[2] This may have helped Hooke to review the financial position, and to form his policy for fulfilling his responsibilities. Despite an attempt to discredit him, there was no discovery of corruption, and any shortfall of money had come about by the increase in the sums distributed to the residents. The master tried to achieve what the Founder had laid down, that expenditure should be less than income, so that a reserve should accumulate for repairs and other changes. In 1846 the payments to the brothers and sisters were kept at their recent level, but by the end of 1847, the master was owed £122.9.2½d. Bank stock worth £300 was sold, and the weekly pay was reduced from six shillings to 4/9d. Jackman sisters had a reduction of three pence, to four shillings. The other sources of income made sure that they always received more than this, and from 1848 to 1853 the average figures were 6/1½d, Jackman sisters 4/5d. Hooke also was strict in observing regulations, noting absences, insisting on dead pay following vacancies, exacting fines for missing chapel. The payment for a gaudy (the name was revived in 1850) was reduced from £1.2s to ten shillings.

The master tried to explain that these reforms were for the benefit of the hospital and its community, but the residents thought most about the immediate loss of cash. Aided by

Abbot's Hospital Guildford

a mischievous outsider, a letter was sent on 3 February 1853 to the Archbishop of Canterbury, J.B. Sumner, as Visitor, signed by the vice-master, William Tidy, with the marks of seven brothers. They complained of the master, "whose venality equals that of the late Master, who instead of taking the Charter and Statutes for his guide, perverts as best suits his own purpose our best guide, and is determined to do so unless a restraint is put on him". They claimed that he threatened to reduce the weekly payments to the half crown provided by George Abbot. The complaint was not only unjustified but too late, for the Visitor's powers had been suspended.

On 10 March 1852 the Court of Chancery issued a decree ordering an enquiry into the endowments of the hospital and the manufacture. The management of the estates was to be reformed to meet modern conditions, and the system of renewing low rents and exacting fines on new leases was to cease. There should be a fair apportioning of income between the hospital and the manufacture. In order to do this the Master of the Court could override the charter and statutes on "mere side-issues", and the Archbishop's powers as Visitor were taken away for the time of the enquiry. A point was made that quitrents for encroachments, such as the building of outhouses by neighbours against the hospital walls, had not been collected for thirty years. Payment was demanded, and from 1853 brought in two shillings a year. The enquiries continued until 1857, but Hooke did not see the outcome, for he died on 18 October 1853, always conscientious, but not fully appreciated.

On 19 October George Russell was chosen as master. He was born in 1781, and was a nephew of Samuel Russell, an earlier master, his father William being Samuel's brother. For the whole of his time, Russell, who had worked in the family bookselling and printing business, had none of the freedom that his predecessors had enjoyed. For the first four years he was controlled by the Court of Chancery, and for the next four years the Charity Commissioners were conducting an enquiry and preparing a new scheme of management, which came into effect less than a month after he died.

On 21 October, two days after Russell took office, the Mayor, William Taylor, Mark Smallpeice, W. Piggott and W. Hooke met the master and vice-master "to examine into the Late Master's accounts and the inventory of the rooms &c". A minute book of hospital business was kept by the master from this time; with enquiries being conducted from outside, there must be no doubt about what was transacted by the hospital. It shews how Russell tried to keep the hospital solvent and efficient. Four days later the master met a commissoner from the Court of Chancery in Mark Smallpeice's office, and received instructions. The master was to receive the same payment as before, but not the annual sum of £8.10.8d allowance for the loss of rooms to the Jackman sisters. When Jackman sisters died they were not to be replaced.

On 26 June 1854 "the Bounds were walked", to examine the outside walls of the hospital, so that quitrents could be charged. This became an annual performance, and led to much bickering as years went by. On 22 July 1854 the cellar under the hall was let for £3

The Reformed Community

a year. On 28 November the hall itself was let for eight months in the year for an evening school. The charge of £10 was to be divided among the brothers and sisters.

The purchase of new gowns in 1845, 1856, 1858 and 1860 indicates that they were still the everyday dress of the residents. Discipline remained an occasional problem. In August 1854 Russell had statutes 8 ("Of honest conversation") and 9 ("What Crimes are to be avoyded, & uppon what Penalties") printed, and a copy put into the room of every brother and sister.

Towards the end of 1854 an exchange of part of the hospital land at Merrow with F. Apted was agreed and sealed. Boundary changes and the sale or exchange of parts of the farms happened from time to time, but after this instance it took place only with the approval of the Charity Commissioners.

In 1856 the lease of Mereden farm at Dorking expired. By the old system it would have been renewed at the same rent (£40) for twenty-one years, on the payment of a £500 fine. By the 1852 Chancery order no fine was to be imposed, and the lease was renewed with the annual rent at £130 for twenty-one years. The hospital's income was in this way increased. Although the residents lost their share of the fine, they were at that time benefitted by the sale of timber at Merrow. Repairs to the farms were infrequent under Russell, but nonetheless the hospital was overdrawn by more than £20 every year until 1859.

In February 1857 the Inspector of Charities, F.O. Martin, paid several visits to Guildford, to enquire into the running of the hospital, to study the accounts, and to visit the sisters. Three brothers took the opportunity to lay complaints against the master, but to no avail. On 30 September 1859 elections were held. W. Chitty was chosen as vice-master, and sisters were appointed as cleaners and nurses. This was repeated on 1 October 1860, when Chitty was again elected. In November a brother was expelled after two previous admonitions, for intoxication and irregular conduct. On 20 June 1861 George Heather was admitted as a brother - the last to be sworn under the Founder's statutes. Three weeks later, on 11 July, the Act of Parliament was passed for the regulation of the hospital.

The Charity Commissioners' 8th Report, 26 February 1861, contained a scheme of management for the hospital, and this was confirmed by the Act. The new regulations[3] were considerably shorter than the Founder's statutes. There were no detailed rules for daily life, and nothing was said about attendance at chapel or Holy Trinity Church. The qualification for appointment as master, and for admission to the hospital remained the same, though when candidates for places could not be found in the ancient borough, they might be accepted from the municipal borough. This clause has led to the extension of the area of benefit through successive boundary changes, including the great enlargement of 1974. The oaths taken on admission were discontinued. The complement of residents was fixed at twenty, normally twelve brothers and eight sisters. Their weekly payment was to be not more than eight shillings, but at times when resources were reduced, admissions might be suspended so that the payments did not fall below five shillings.

Abbot's Hospital Guildford

The greatest change was the dissolution of the corporate existence of the master, brethren and sisters[4], and the creation of a board of Governors to manage the hospital. Nine Governors were official – the Mayor, the Rectors of Holy Trinity and St Mary, St Nicolas' and Stoke-next-Guildford, the master of the Grammar School, and the two senior aldermen and two senior councillors,[5] these four to be members of the Church of England. Four non-official Governors were to be chosen from residents of the town, or within seven miles of it. In the first instance they were to be appointed by the Charity Commission with the concurrence of the Archbishop of Canterbury. Vacancies in these places were to be filled by election by the board, and approved by the Commissioners and the Archbishop. The estates of the hospital were now vested in the Governors, and investments were to be transferred to the Official Trustees of Charitable Funds, to be held as part of the hospital's endowment. Provision was made for the division between the hospital and Archbishop Abbot's School, and this was effected in 1867.[6]

The Governors were responsible for appointing the master, but must not do so within six weeks of the vacancy occurring. The Archbishop's endorsement of the appointment was needed. He was to be paid £70 a year, with a coal allowance of £5. Brothers and sisters were appointed by the Governors, from applications received by the master. One of the brothers might be appointed vice-master, by the Governors, and paid £4 a year. The sisters no longer had to undertake nursing duties. The Archbishop was not stated to be the Visitor of the hospital, but that relationship was implied by the need to refer to him for approval. The income of the charity was to be used to pay thirty shillings a year to the Rector of Holy Trinity, as before, and to repair and insure the hospital and other buildings, and to meet necessary outgoings and expenses.

Following the Charitable Trusts Act of 1853, charities throughout the country were obliged to conform to new regulations. There was most dislocation when curruption or inefficiency was revealed, and there was greater continuity when those in responsible positions retained their offices. At Croydon a new scheme of management for Whitgift's Hospital was approved by the Court of Chancery on 29 March 1855. John Pimm was warden at least by 1854, when he was described by one of the brothers as barely literate. "He can only just write his own name."[7] Nonetheless he was still in office in 1861. At Guildford there was no such continuity. On 9 August 1861, before the governing body was constituted, George Russell died, and was buried in the family vault in Holy Trinity churchyard. The hospital was without a master for the unprecedented period of eleven and a half weeks.

On 2 September, a Charity Commission order named the Governors. The official Governors were John Palmer the Mayor, Thomas Ludham, Rector of Holy Trinity and St Mary since 1851, Thomas Goodwin Hatchard, Rector of St Nicolas' since 1856, Richard Shepherd, Rector of Stoke since 1858, Dr Henry Gordon Merriman, master of the Grammar School since 1859; the two senior aldermen were Thomas Jenner Sells and Henry Piper, and the two senior councillors William Smith and Jesse Boxall. The four Governors appointed by the Charity Commission were Sir George Shaw-Lefevre of

The Reformed Community

Sutton Place, Arthur Pooley Onslow of Send Grove, James More-Molyneux of Loseley and Ross Donnelly Mangles of Guildford.[8]

The Governors met for the first time on 16 September, and from the outset it was plain that they intended to *govern*. John Palmer, the Mayor, took the chair, and that remained the custom for nearly a century; only Shaw-Lefevre and Hatchard were absent. The Act of Parliament containing the scheme was read. A survey and valuation of the Ewhurst property was ordered, as the lease was due for renewal. The appointment of master was to be advertised, and posters were printed, signed by W.H. & M. Smallpeice, who acted as solicitors for the hospital.

The Governors met again on 28 September. A committee consisting of Ludham, Onslow and Shaw-Lefevre was appointed to draw up "Regulations for the conduct of the Hospital". William Tidy was appointed vice-master. The choice of a master was deferred, and was considered at the next meeting, on 12 October, when Hatchard was present. Three names were proposed: the Reverend John Richards, who had worked in Guildford since 1820, and had been chaplain of the Guildford Union since 1838, was proposed by Sells and seconded by Ludham; William Russell, formerly a soldier, and brother of the last master, was proposed by Boxall and seconded by Smith: Thomas Terry was proposed by Palmer and seconded by Piper. Terry was the successful candidate. The Archbishop of Canterbury, J.B. Sumner, wrote to give his approval, and Terry was installed on 28 October, at noon.

The emphasis on government by Governors was made plain straight away. The new master was not invited to their meetings, and the Governors made the routine decisions that had in the past been within the competence of the master, or the master and the brethren. It was they who expelled Thomas Smallpeice in December 1861 for persistent drunkenness, in accordance with the new statutes.

In November the Governors decided to appoint a clerk and receiver, who would be paid £30 *per annum* to look after the business affairs of the hospital. Mark Smallpeice was chosen for this post, and was instructed to "procure the requisite Books and Box for the same and order a Bell for the Board Room". The weekly payment to the brothers and sisters was immediately fixed at five shillings. To ease acceptance of the new rules, an extra payment of fifteen shillings was made to each of them in November, "in lieu of the division that has taken place at this time" in the past. Careful management made it possible for the weekly payment to be raised to six shillings in 1865.

The Governors looked for ways to improve their income. In November 1861 the upper hall was let to Mr Harding for a singing class on Tuesday and Friday evenings, for £1 a quarter. In 1862 Mr Shillingford asked for a seven-year lease of the stable and coach house for £6. It was advertised, and Mr Strudwick was given the lease for £7 *per annum*, in 1864. Later, in 1871, it was decided that Gates might use the cellars under the chapel for £5 *per annum*. In 1869 the Governors were sufficiently confident to ask the Charity

Abbot's Hospital Guildford

Commission for permission to increase the number of sisters by two. This was granted, and the extra women were to be received on the same terms as the rest.

The main source of income remained the endowment farms, and changes in that area will be dealt with later. Smallpeice's first statement was for fifteen months, 29 September 1861- 31 December 1862. The first statement for a calendar year was for 1863, and it is given as an example of the funding of the charity, and its expenses at the beginning of the modern period.

Receipts		Payments	
Balance at banker 58. 7. 4		Weekly pay to Bros &	
due to Master 3.14. 4	54. 13. 00	Sisters inc. extra pay to the sick	266. 2. 6
Yrs rent from Merriden	125. 2. 6	Master's salary 70	
1½ yr Merrow Farm	102. 8. 9	coal allowance 5	75. 0. 0
yr Salthurst	12. 0. 0	Vice Master	6. 0. 0
2 yrs Rumbeams	108. 10. 0	Clerk & receiver	30. 0. 0
1 yr Woolpits	35. 0. 0	Rates, taxes, Gas, insurance	
		Quit rents	18. 8. 3
½ Yr Highlands less tax	19. 5. 0	tradesmen's bills inc. £32.4	
		for cloth for cloaks & gowns	76. 19. 4
W. Wantley annuity less tax	12. 0. 8		472. 10. 1
Dividend on Molineux charity	59. 19. 10	Abp. Abbot's School	
Official Trustees of		Merriden	
Charitable Trust	87. 5. 8	Salthurst ⅓ rents	29. 7. 8
	616. 5. 5	Merrow	
rent for cellar	3. 0. 0	Woolpits	
		Gardener	4. 18. 11
	619. 5. 5	for tenants' dinners	1. 0. 0
		balance at bank 95.15. 7	
		in Master's hands 12.11. 4	108. 6. 11
			619. 5. 5
			(sic)

Hospital discipline seems not to have caused many problems in these years. Absences from chapel were noted in the journal. In 1863 the master was given authority to permit brothers and sisters to attend Sunday evening services, provided they were back by half past eight. In 1873 the Governors resolved that a notice should be printed and put up in the men's rooms, warning them against pocketing tips for shewing people the building, instead of putting the money into the box. This fault would make the brothers 'liable to dismissal'.

The Reformed Community

William Tidy was still vice-master when he died in March 1866. In April William Chitty was chosen to succeed him. In 1868 Chitty was dismissed because he had misappropriated coal. Trimmer and Hatchard, the Rectors of Holy Trinity and St Nicolas', were deputed to choose a successor, and William Birch was appointed in February. Birch died on 11 September 1880. By his will, made in 1872, he left £100 to the hospital, the first bequest from a brother or sister of which there is record. The income was "to be once in every year applied for the benefit of the brothers and sisters of the aforesaid Trinity Hospital either to enable them to dine together or to be divided equally between them".[9]

In 1864 the Governors decided that it was desirable for the hospital to have a resident nurse. The Charity Commission's approval was sought, but there was a delay. In January 1865 a further application was made; a nurse was "considered indispensable to the humane treatment of the very old and helpless inmates". In the meanwhile the master was instructed to visit all the rooms daily, and to go to the sick more often than that. In March the Commission sent approval for the appointment of a nurse, to be paid not more than seven shillings a week, and allowed to occupy a room. In 1872 the Governors made the additional provision for paid assistance for the nurse, whenever there was "extreme illness of any of the Brethren or Sisters". In 1866 the Governors applied for permission to appoint a medical officer. In July approval was received. A doctor might be paid £20 *per annum*, that sum to include the cost of medicine and appliances. The Governors appointed one of themselves, T.J. Sells, as the first medical officer.

In 1867 the appointment of a chaplain to the hospital was considered, and it was suggested that the annual payment should be £60. In 1868 the proposal was reviewed, and the lower sum of £40 was agreed. The Rector of Holy Trinity, R.W. Trimmer, was prepared to accept the position for that stipend. It may be wondered why it was thought necessary for a community of about two dozen, living across the road from a parish church which they attended regularly, to have a chaplain. The reason is probably found in the poor endowment of the united benefice of Holy Trinity and St Mary at that time, only £248, compared with Stoke, £597, and St Nicolas, £600. Payment for the chaplaincy would provide a welcome augmentation. The Charity Commissioners did not approve of the proposal, but allowed the payment of not more than £10 "to a clergyman .... upon condition of his giving such spiritual ministrations to the Alms-people as they may from time to time require". The Governors persevered in their request, but the refusal was maintained. Furthermore, the Commissioners observed that the requirement of daily attendance in chapel for divine service "would introduce a religious element into the administration of the Charity which is not contemplated by the recent Statutory Scheme and appears indeed to be opposed to its design". In May 1869 Trimmer accepted the £10 nomination, on the terms that had been allowed. He was straight away described as the chaplain, as was his successor at Holy Trinity in 1882, F.E. Tower, and the term has been in general use ever since. In 1869 a surplice was bought for use in the chapel.

Abbot's Hospital Guildford

The northern boundary wall of the lower garden was replaced with an iron fence in 1862. This was moved in 1868 when the Local Government Board paid £10 to the Governors for a narrow strip of land, to widen North Street.

By June 1862 a house committee had been formed, to be responsible for the upkeep of the building and its grounds. In August 1882 the Governors suggested to the committee that when rooms were vacant, they should be decorated with wallpaper, instead of white-wash. In 1883 the committee was authorised to put the quadrangle "into a proper state" and keep it so. Later that year the committee was charged with seeing to the repair of the two northern chimneys. The tall chimneys continued to give trouble, and were dealt with in the large-scale restoration a few years later. The lower garden was rarely mentioned in the minutes and journal. In 1864 the committee reported that there was a contract with Messrs A. Hart and Son to crop and keep in order the vegetable garden for £7.10s *per annum*, and to supply plants for the flower garden, and keep it in order for £6.10s. In 1882 new gooseberry and currant bushes were planted, to replace the old ones. So the garden was still expected to produce some food for the residents.

In 1866 a letter was received from the South Kensington Museum, referring to a proposed exhibition of historical portraits. The clerk was instructed to "write and state that there are no portraits in the possession of the Governors" - with little regard to truth.

It was soon discovered that the aging hospital buildings needed more than occasional repairs. In April 1867 the Governors decided that window repairs were urgently required. The mullions were to be made good, and the small panes and iron bars were to be replaced with plate glass, both in the courtyard and on the High Street front. The *Surrey Advertiser* welcomed this decision, which, it said, would improve the appearance, "& make more lightsome & pleasing the appartments of the Inmates". The Governors very soon became alarmed at the likely cost of what they were undertaking, and called in the Guildford architect Henry Woodyer to make a report and recommendations. It was received, and considered on 5 June. It revealed that much must be done. The stonework was in poor condition, the windows and stringcourses especially, and Woodyer suggested that the chalk should be replaced with Bath stone. Parts of the parapets needed to be rebuilt, and some of the walls repointed, especially where there had been settlement. Copings needed to be reset, and in some places renewed. The roof timbers and tiles were in generally good condition, but in the chapel the tie beams had been cut out, causing bulges in the walls and harm to the windows. Woodyer's estimate for the repairs was £1259.7.4d.

The Governors accepted the architect's advice, which included leaving the small panes in the windows. After competitive tender, W. and T. Smith were appointed as contractors. Work began during the winter, and continued until the autumn of 1872, orders being given to Smiths as money became available. The repairs to the windows, and the introduction of Bath stone came early in the programme. The cost for all these repairs was £1477.16.7d. A second programme lasted from 1874 to 1876, concerned more with the exterior of the north range, and this cost £379.4.6d.

The Reformed Community

Samuel Russell's bell turret needed repair. It was decided that it should be replaced with one to Woodyer's design, and this was in position by March 1871. Smith's estimate for it was £97.17s. Woodyer believed that the terrace and steps leading to the garden had been added to the building, and he considered that they did harm to the structure, causing wet to penetrate the basement and foundations. It appears that lavatory accommodation had been provided near to these steps, and Woodyer wanted all this to be removed, and some other way of going to the garden arranged. In July 1871 the Governors decided that the terrace, steps and lavatories must remain. Two and a half years later the master was given a lavatory in his own lodgings.

There were other improvements. In 1870 gas lights were fitted in all six staircases. They were lit and extinguished by the gas company for a daily charge of one penny. The paths in the quadrangle were laid out and edged with ornamental brick. All the staircases were fitted with bells, so that the residents could "communicate with each other in case of illness during the night". A box for their letters was put up near the master's lodgings in 1875. For those who wanted to use it, a hip bath was bought in 1881, for £2.0.3d.

Repairs to Holy Trinity Church were carried out under Woodyer's supervision in 1869. The Governors contributed £15 for renewing the seats that the brothers and sisters occupied, and £7 for repairs to the founder's tomb.

The Governors found that they had increasingly to take account of their responsibilities as landlords, and as years passed, parts of the historic endowment estates were sold, or exchanged for other land. In December 1863 a parliamentary notice was received, stating the intention of running the Guildford to Leatherhead railway through the hospital land at Merrow. In 1866 the Rector of Merrow, H.A. Bowles, asked to exchange some land at the corner of Boxgrove Road for the hospital's Hall Deane field, so that he could build a house there. It was agreed that the exchange should take place, the Rector paying the costs, and also £70 for standing timber. It was also agreed that the Rector and church wardens of Merrow should buy not more than a quarter of an acre of hospital land to enlarge the churchyard, for twenty guineas, the purchasers to pay the expenses, and for reinstating the wall, cartshed and pond. This sale was completed by February 1868.

Property held at a distance was not easy to keep under view, and it could be abused. In 1864 there was the annoyance that there was an encroachment at Highlands farm Horsham, where a broom-maker called Dewdney had enclosed part of the frontage. Enquiries were made, and in 1866 the clerk was instructed to take steps to eject him. In 1866 the Governors were notified that the London to Worthing railway would pass through their land at Horsham. In 1870 a donation of £10 was sent to the Vicar of Horsham for increasing the number of school places there.

As leases ended, the possibility of sale rather than renewal was considered. In 1877 an offer was received for Mereden farm at Dorking, but the price was not high enough, and a lease for seven years was granted. In the same year part of Hornbrook farm was offered to Barclay Sandeman for £1500, and the valuation of the timber. The sale was

Abbot's Hospital Guildford

approved by the Charity Commission, and it was completed early in 1878. The price received was £1582.7.6d, and this was invested by the Charity Commissioners in £1644.0.6d consols. This was the first stage in the significant disposal of the founder's endowments. In 1872 the proprietor of the West Wantley estate asked to buy the rent charge of £12.10s. No offer was recorded, and the Governors declined to sell it.

Woolpits farm at Ewhurst, bought by the hospital in 1768, was the first larger property for which a sale was considered. A request to purchase it was rejected in 1864. In 1882 another opportunity came, and it was sold to Henry Doulton of the Lambeth Potteries for £5000, and £496.12.1d for the valuation of the timber. Three per cent consols were bought, £5503.9.9d for £5496.12.1d. *The West Surrey Times* of 28 February 1885 used this as an example of good management. The farm had produced an annual rent of £35; the invested proceeds of the sale brought in £150. The remaining farms should therefore be sold, the newspaper advised. The short-term advantage was plain, but no-one could forecast the range of property values in succeeding years.

In 1877 the Governors began to consider an exchange of land with Lord Onslow.[10] Several pieces of hospital land at Merrow and Send, amounting to over 110 acres, were given and in return the Governors received eighty-six acres at Stoughton, Shepherd's farm. This was completed in 1880. Shepherd's farm proved a source of much trouble to the Governors, who for many years had to deal with sick tenants, and disputes about access, boundaries, buildings and drains.

In 1879 Dr Sells resigned as medical officer, because of ill health. He was succeeded by his son, Dr Charles John Sells. In 1884 Mark Smallpeice, who had served as clerk to the Governors since 1861, was elected a non-official Governor. He was succeeded as clerk by Humphrey Percy Smallpeice, his son.

The new way in which the hospital's affairs were managed is illustrated significantly by the absence of any reference to the master personally in the preceding fifteen paragraphs. Thomas Terry, who had been master since 1861, seems to have been of a retiring disposition, and towards the end of his long period in office, he became more or less invisible. In 1878 the Governors asked the Charity Commission whether a pension might be given to the master, whose age was causing him to find the work difficult; but Terry declined to discuss this subject. In April 1880 the Governors decided to discuss his inefficiency, "arising from age and infirmity" at their next meeting, but when the time came they could not think what to do. In January 1883 the practice was begun of signing the master's journal by the chairman of the Governors at their meetings. By this time pencil lines were ruled in the journal to assist Terry in his writing, as his hand was shaky and his sight failing. By June 1884, the master had been ill for two years. The exasperated Governors, meeting in the boardroom, only a few feet from his sick-bed, made an allowance to the vice-master, Philip Hyde, in recognition of the extra work that fell to him. The accounts were kept by the master's granddaughter, and in February 1885 a deficiency of £19 was found. The Governors said that it must be made good, or the sum would be deducted from Terry's pay. Thomas Terry died at midnight 20-21

The Reformed Community

February 1885. He was buried in the new Mount cemetery on 26 February. The residents followed his coffin to the foot of the Mount, but did not attempt to climb the hill.

The time of waiting for the mastership to be vacant gave opportunity for thought about the future. On 28 February the *Surrey Advertiser* suggested that the scheme should be altered to allow a "man and his wife, who will be better able than a single individual to look after the wants of the inmates". The *Surrey Times* of the same date said that the master should be "an educated man of good business capacity and some energy, and he should be not much over fifty". The paper made other suggestions for reform, which will be noted later. On 6 March the Governors resolved to write to the Charity Commission enquiring whether in future a master might be removed if he were found incapable through age or infirmity, and given an allowance for life. The Commission did not allow a standing arrangement of this kind, but pointed out that the removal of an incapacitated master could be achieved under a section of the Charitable Trusts Act 1853.

In the meanwhile the Governors had advertised the vacancy in the local newspapers. There were three applicants, from whom, on 17 March, George Challen was unanimously chosen. He was in business in the High Street as a tailor, draper and hatter. He took up residence on 27 April, and Archbishop Benson's approval was received soon afterwards.

The West Surrey Times encouraged the Governors to introduce a daily common meal, to be eaten in the common hall, with the master presiding. This would be of especial benefit to the men, who were not used to cooking, and often ate bread and cheese at an inn. The one good meal should be provided free, and a cook would be needed. The paper also suggested that out-pensioners should be elected, and given a weekly allowance until vacant rooms were available for them. The additional cost of these reforms could be met by selling more land, and reference was made to the sale of Woolpits farm, and the benefit that that had brought in increased income. The paper returned to the subject on 20 February 1886, calling the Governors a "very respectable, but very antiquated and stolid body". The landed property was "dormant wealth", and the income could be more than doubled if the farms were sold. The suggestion was not accepted, and in 1889 some of the residents asked permission to eat together in the hall on weekdays, each paying threepence a day. Permission was not given, but it was decided that the hall should be open from 5 to 9.30 p.m. in the winter for "social intercourse". £20.8s was spent furnishing it.

In 1887 Queen Victoria's golden jubilee was celebrated with a dinner costing £11.6.2d. Another social event seems to have started in 1889, an annual feast or "gala day" early in the year, paid for by voluntary subscriptions. Before the 1890 feast the Governors decided that visitors should leave by 9 o'clock, and that the feast must end by 10.

The walking of the bounds became associated with Ascension Day in Challen's time, and the quitrents were collected from the neighbours. F.E. Tower died early in 1885, and was succeded as Rector of Holy Trinity by Arthur Sutton Valpy, who was appointed as chaplain to the hospital on 29 May.

Abbot's Hospital Guildford

The duties of the nurse were not properly defined, and they were specified in 1885. After this, the nurse, Mrs Lewis, was not found competent, and she was dismissed. The appointment was advertised in some local and national newspapers. *The West Surrey Times* on 17 July 1886 commented that the Governors offered "the munificent sum of 12s a week, without rations. A ridiculous salary for the services required." Mrs Lavinia Donellan was appointed.

Regard for the comfort of the residents led to some improvements. In 1886 it was decided that when rooms fell vacant they should be furnished with carpets, bed and bedding. Iron bedsteads were provided, each with a straw palliasse and a flock bed. In 1887 gas was laid on to all the rooms.

From 1885 there were discussions about increasing the accommodation of the hospital. In May that year the architect W.G. Lower suggested alterations to the storerooms below the north range, so that rooms could be formed there. The Governors asked for a scheme that would use the stable for this purpose. Lower produced one, and was then asked for another, using the large room over the hall. When he submitted that, in July, the Governors, on the suggestion of the Rector of St Nicolas', W.S. Sanders, decided to defer considering it until a committee had investigated the state of the buildings. The plan to use the stable was ruled out in 1887, when it was repaired at a cost of £81.9.6d, and let to R. Porter as a dry store, for an annual rent of £10. Valpy, the Rector of Holy Trinity, raised the question of extra rooms again in 1890, and it was referred to the house committee.

Henry Woodyer was asked to report on the building, and was paid three guineas for his report in 1888. He said that the stonework of the chapel windows, which was chalk, was in bad condition. To repair the mullions and sills would cost between £70 and £80. it was decided that only the mullions should be dealt with.

Holy Trinity Church was enlarged to the designs of A.W. Blomfield in 1887-8. The Governors paid for the cleaning and restoring of Abbot's tomb, and its removal to the newly formed south transept. This cost £50. A further £39.10s was spent on iron railings to surround the tomb, designed by Blomfield and made by the local foundry, Filmer and Mason in 1889.

There was another sale of land, the Mark of Merrow, in 1890. The proceeds, £3000, were used to buy £3080.7.5d $2^3/_4$% consols.

On 10 April 1890 the master, George Challen, died suddenly. After taking prayers he worked as usual, and then went into the quadrangle to advise some residents not to stay out in the cold. He returned to his lodging and died in his chair.

There were seven applicants for the mastership, and the Governors chose Henry Harris, elected on 23 May 1890. He moved into his lodgings on 19 June, a fortnight before Archbishop Benson's approval was received. Harris was an old boy of the Bluecoat School, and had worked as an employed builder. His skill was useful to the hospital, as

The Reformed Community

was his keenness for gardening. His wife had died in 1889, and for some of the time at least, his daughter made her home with him at the hospital.

Harris was master for a long time, until 1913. They were mostly uneventful years, though the peace of the community was sometimes disturbed by the master's tendency to be querulous; and there were unproved doubts of his honesty. There was a tragedy in 1891, when Mrs Rule was found dead, with her clothes burning, and Harris advised all the brothers and sisters who had no fireguards to acquire them. In 1892 Mrs Donellan wished to resign from the position of nurse, because of Harris's attitude to her. He was called before the Governors, and said that "owing to her unsociable manner they had been unable to agree of late". They were both told to try harder, and she agreed to stay. The nurse was told to make her daily report to the master at 10.30 a.m. The nurse resigned in 1894 after a disagreement over her duties. Her successor, Mrs Emily Eldershaw, complained that Harris treated her more like a servant than a nurse, but the Governors found her generally unsatisfactory, and asked her to leave. Two more nurses in succession resigned because of their inability to work happily with Harris, and one complained of interference by his daughter.

Henry Harris set out to be a friendly master. His early weeks were made difficult by the hostility of one of the brothers, J.B. Hicks, who was disruptive and defiant, and very often drunk. He was expelled in 1892. On 23 December 1890, for example, there was a pre-Christmas dinner. Two turkeys were given by Colonel Godwin Austen. Harris gave a piece of beef, and "a little Beer & tobacco, and [they] made themselves very comfortable, round the fire on the hearth". He tried to increase the social activities of the hospital, both by his own efforts and encouraging others. On 6 July 1893 a dinner was held to mark the marriage of the Duke of York and Princess Mary of Teck. Flags were used to decorate the hospital on this occasion. Queen Victoria's diamond jubilee was celebrated very thoroughly on 16 September 1897. After a hot dinner, with the Mayor, Christopher Wrist, in the chair, the community set out in three brakes and pairs through Clandon Park, where they were shewn rooms in the house. At the Railway Hotel at Horsley they were given wine and biscuits, and then they went on to Wisley for tea. There were more refreshments when they returned to the hospital at about 7 o'clock. "The Inmates said they enjoyed themselves very much and had never had such a treat before." Winter comfort was not increased however, when the Governors rejected the request for a fire in the hall in the winter months. A modern note appeared with the coronation of King George V in 1911. As well as an expenditure of £26.10s on illuminations, catering and flags, it was recorded that Mr Puttock "invited the Inmates & Staff, to the Picture Palace, 21 went and enjoyed themselves very much, Carriage provided to take the feeble ones to and fro". Two years later another aspect of modern life presented a threat. In May 1913 the house committee reported that they had closed the gates to visitors because "Suffragettes had recently visited the Hospital and obtained certain information with reference thereto". The Governors endorsed the committee's action, and no visitors were admitted until September, when they were limited to six at a time, always accompanied by a brother. This restriction was removed in September 1914, when the outbreak of war had diverted the women's energies to other activities.

The place of the chapel in the life of the hospital was altered considerably while Harris was master. From the beginning it had been used for daily prayers, the furnishings being suitable for that purpose. For the sacraments, the master, brothers and sisters crossed to Holy Trinity Church. In 1891 the Governors approved the spending of not more than £15 on a communion table and rail for the chapel. The cost rose to £20. On 2 December 1891, the Reverend H.C. Gaye, curate at Holy Trinity, celebrated the eucharist in the chapel, with twenty communicants.[11] From this time the eucharist was normally celebrated once a month, usually by a curate. Valpy applied to the Bishop of Winchester for a licence for the chapel to be used for the eucharist, and this was received in 1892. The fee was £1.11s. Other fittings and liturgical ornaments were acquired, including a harmonium given by the Mayoress, Mrs Wells, linen, cruets and candlesticks. An old chalice was given by Valpy in 1894, believed to be early Jacobean.[12] In 1895 Valpy resigned the rectory and chaplaincy, and was succeeded by C.F. Grant, who in turn was succeeded by E.C. Kirwan in 1907.

From 1890 additional devotions took place in the chapel. A Sunday afternoon service was begun, conducted by Mr Ball, and Miss Beck played a borrowed harmonium. Occasionally choirboys from Holy Trinity or St Mary's were brought in. This voluntary lay leadership did not last long. After a while a weekday morning service with an address was instituted, about once a month, conducted by the Rector or a curate. In 1896 Grant held the first part of the funeral of one of the sisters, Mrs Dalman, in the chapel. Afterwards the brothers and sisters followed the coffin to the entrance archway. This practice was repeated from time to time.

In July 1890, the Governors decided that the need for increased accommodation had been proved, but agreed to take no measures to achieve it until £1000 had accumulated to make it possible. The Governors also considered the way in which their own business was conducted. In July 1891 it was announced that the Charity Commission had approved the regulations that had been proposed. The Mayor of Guildford was to be chairman at meetings if he was present, otherwise the meeting should elect a chairman. The quorum for meetings was to be five Governors. The chairman was given a second or casting vote. Resolutions were to be binding on all Governors, and might be altered or rescinded only at a meeting with special notice given. General meetings must be at intervals of not more than two months, with at least three days' notice. The clerk might call a special meeting when there was need, and when there was a vacancy in the hospital. There might be committees for special purposes.

In 1900 a consequence of the division of the borough into wards was dealt with. The Charity Commission approved of a variation of the scheme, to provide that when more than two senior councillors were members of the Church of England, the Council should decide each year which of them its representative Governors should be. In 1901 Mark

The Reformed Community

Smallpeice died, and was followed as a Governor by his son, Humphrey Smallpeice, the clerk. Alfred Portsmouth was appointed clerk in his place.

After the repairs that had been carried out to the buildings by the Governors during the masterships of Terry and Challen, not much was needed while Harris was master. In 1891 Filmer and Mason made new weather vanes for the gatehouse, costing £24.9s. In 1901 the works of the clock were taken away for repair by Salsburys, because it "dont Strike regular". In 1910 the house committee began to consider two matters of improvements. The Inspector of Nuisances had written to say that the number of lavatories was inadequate. The Guildford Electricity Supply Company had suggested that electric light should be introduced into the hospital. In 1913 five chimneys were repaired, with care taken to match the old bricks. In the garden apple trees were planted in 1894, for both cooking and keeping apples. Unsatisfactory pear trees were removed in 1907. In that year the Borough Council asked for a change in the line of the northern boundary, as part of a road-widening scheme. With the consent of the Charity Commission and the Board of Agriculture and Fisheries, this took place in 1908. In 1913 it was decided that invitations to tender for the care of the hospital gardens should be made only to members of the Church of England.

The management of the hospital's estates during these years required more attention and care. The farms brought in a steady but small rent, and produced timber for repairs, but opportunities for sale were taken. The first sale in this period was a quarter of an acre for the enlargement of Merrow churchyard. This was completed in 1892, and the proceeds, £200, were used to buy £205.7.10d consols for £199.14.10d (commission 5/2d). In 1893 H.J. Burkitt approached the Governors with the request to purchase land at Shepherd's farm to provide a site for a church at Stoughton. In 1897 the land was sold for £200, and £177.19.6d consols bought for £199.15.6d (commission 4/6d). In 1904 a further small strip of ground was also sold to Emmanuel Church for £64.1.3d, and £70.6s consols were bought for £63.19.6d (commission 1/9d). In 1898 the sale of Mereden farm at Dorking was discussed. It was mostly wood and rough land, and the Governors were willing to sell it for £10,000. The Charity Commissioners insisted that the price should not be less than £11,000. This was received in 1899, and invested in £9932.5.7d consols, bought for £10,987.11.8d (commission £1.4.2d). In 1904 the Guildford Union bought eight acres of Shepherd's farm for £2000, and the Governors bought £2250.7s consols for £1997.3.9d (commission £2.16.3d). New tenancies began in 1904 at Hall Place Merrow for £85 *per annum*, and at the remainder of Shepherd's farm for £90 *per annum*.

In 1906 investments were sold to pay for the building of a new farmhouse at Highlands farm Horsham, and to convert the old house into two cottages. The cost was £1083.15s, and the Charity Commission ordered that this sum should be reinvested within twenty years.[13] The same condition was imposed in 1908 when £791.5s was spent on building new cowsheds at Shepherd's farm. The payments from West Wantley farm were received very irregularly. In 1912 arrears of £87.10s were recorded.

Abbot's Hospital Guildford

Despite the increased revenue when farms were sold and the proceeds invested, the Governors found it difficult to pay for all the expenses out of their income. This was partly due to the cost of repairs to the farm properties, which the rents and the sale of timber did not meet. In 1905 the revenue from Hall Place farm at Merrow was £90, and expenses amounted to £67.17.6d. In 1906 the revenue had risen to £100, but the expenses were £121.11.1d. To meet a crisis in 1906, an overdraft was arranged with the Capital and Counties Bank for not more than £350. A month later this was discharged when timber had been sold for £325.17.6d.

In 1892 the insurance cover of the hospital was increased from £5000 to £9800, and the stable from £100 to £200. In 1893 the furniture and fittings of the hospital were insured for £1000. These figures were the same in 1901, when the cover for the farms was noted: Highlands £960, Hornbrook £215, Rumbeams £1400, Shepherd's £1250.

By 1904 bicycling had become very popular, and country people were riding into the town and some were parking their machines in the small front yard and under the archway. The master was instructed to prevent it. In 1909 the Governors paid Arthur Moon and Sons £34.8s for cleaning and renovating George Abbot's tomb.

Harris continued to try to be a kindly master of the hospital. On Christmas Day 1901 he noted that he and his daughter gave seven of the residents "Christmas dinner, looked after them all day, not having any of their own friend to look after them". But complaints continued, and the house committee had reported to the Governors in 1899 that it had considered representations made by Councillor John Bullen. They concerned such matters as the opening of the almsboxes, the disposal of garden produce, the porter's duties, and the master's attention to sick brothers and sisters, and the language that he sometimes used. The Governors accepted the committee's recommendations, and they were read to the master. No clear complaint was found over the last two issues, no change to be made in the porter's duties. Garden produce was to be divided carefully among the residents, and none was to be taken out of the hospital. The almsboxes had each to be fitted with an extra lock, and the master and vice-master were to have one key to each box. The new locks were fitted before the year was out.

In September 1905 the clerk reported to the Governors that on 24 August he had "found the Master of the Hospital in the Chapel with the entrance door closed and with a key in one of the Poor Boxes in the act of either locking or unlocking such box". The Governors decided that there must be two new iron boxes, one in the chapel and one at the hospital entrance, each with two different locks, the keys to be kept by the master and clerk. The vice-master was relieved of this responsibility as he had been for a long while bed-ridden. The boxes were made by Filmer & Co. In 1910 open war broke out between the master and William Mitchell, one of the brothers. Several times in 1909 Mitchell had been accused of drunkenness. He was disciplined by having his allowance stopped, and he was found not fit to act as porter. In February 1910 Harris accused him of repeated misconduct, and Mitchell counter-attacked by accusing the master of drunkenness, on a

The Reformed Community

day when he had fallen over in the garden. The Governors admonished both men seriously. After further warnings, Mitchell was expelled in July 1910.

Henry Harris died on 20 September 1913, aged 83. He was buried at Stoughton cemetery after a funeral at Holy Trinity. The Governors allowed his family to stay in the lodgings for a fortnight "for the purpose of cleaning &c."

The vacancy was advertised in local newspapers, and on 23 October the Governors considered five applicants. Philip Griggs Palmer was elected. The choice was ratified on 4 November, when the statutory interval after Harris's death had passed, and Palmer moved into the lodgings on 11 November. Three days later he was "formally introduced to the Brethren, Sisters and Nurses by the Clerk. All the inmates assembled in the Dining Hall where the introduction took place." Archbishop Davidson's approval was dated 7 November.

Palmer was born in 1854 and educated at Archbishop Abbot's School, entering as a paying boy in July 1862 end being moved to the free list three months later. When he left school he went to London to learn tailoring. After seven years he returned to Guildford and joined his father's business at 157 High Street, and succeeded him when he died in 1895. Philip Palmer was an active churchman, and took part in the London mission in 1874. By 1888 he had become sacristan at Holy Trinity. Later he became a lay reader, and for more than fifteen years walked to Wood Street to conduct services in a schoolroom. His other interest was history, especially the study of records. In 1886 the Governors had given him permission to look at the archives of the hospital. When he became master he gave much of his spare time to the study of the hospital's history, and made detailed summaries of the registers and accounts.[14]

For the first few months of his mastership, Palmer had to keep his business going, but he disposed of it in March 1914. By then he had already had his telephone moved from his shop to the master's lodgings. As soon as he had time, he began a thorough inspection of the hospital buildings, and used his journal to draw the Governors' attention to defects and needs for improvement. It was not until December 1916 that the Governors decided "to ask the Master into the Meeting of the Governors at the end of each Meeting", a small approach to regarding the master as a partner rather than a servant. Earlier that year the clerk, A. Portsmouth, retired. The post was advertised, with the salary of £25 *per annum*, and F.H. Elsley was chosen from the applicants.

The first world war did not much affect life at the hospital. Palmer was alert to the possibility of attack from the air, and in November 1914 arranged for the light in the quadrangle to be extinguished soon after the gates were closed, "as it renders the building conspicuous from above". There was a little excitement on 1 May 1915, when the hospital was "invaded by successive military cyclist detachments taking part in manoeuvres". In November curtains and blinds were put up to darken the windows of the stairs, buttery and other parts of the building. On 31 March 1916, at 10 o'clock at night, there was a "Police warning of aircraft danger". the Chief Constable sent two St

Abbot's Hospital Guildford

John's Ambulance Corps officers, who stayed by the gate. The nurses stayed up with the master until the recall soon after 3 o'clock in the morning. A similar alert followed on 3 April; the residents were not told. Summer time was introduced in 1916 to create a longer working day, and Palmer noted that the clocks were altered on 21 May. In June 1917 it was announced that Guildford was in "the area of defence against 'Hostile Daylight Air-Raids'" and the Chief Constable made suggestions for the residents' safety. Soon after that there were several daytime alerts. In September a "'take shelter' drill was held, the boys of Abbot's School (105) occupying the inner cellar". This plan was approved by the Governors a month later. On 11 November 1918, when news of the armistice was received, Palmer noted that all possible flags were put out, and that the clock was allowed to strike at night for the first time for four years. On 6 July 1919, a day of thanksgiving for peace, a tea party was held in the common hall.

For practical purposes, the dangers of warfare proved less than risk from neighbouring premises. On 17 June 1916 a fire broke out in Gates's buildings to the east of the hospital. It was noticed at 2.15 a.m. by Edwards, the caretaker of Barclays Bank, who told the police, and by Ray Dalby, the son of the landlord of the Three Pigeons Inn, to which the fire soon spread. Gates's buildings were over two hundred years old, and very fragile, and much inflammable material was stored there. The police called the fire brigade, which arrived in two minutes, under Chief Officer Hickman. Access to fight the fire was difficult, and Hickman called the assistance of the fire force from Dennis's motor works, who came with a powerful engine capable of directing jets of water. Hoses were directed from the roof of Barclays Bank, from a point in the hospital, and from Ram corner in the High Street, the site of the inn demolished in 1913. The fire officers asked for the way into the roof space, but there was no means of entering it. The sheer east wall of the hospital was a barrier to the fire, but there was a fear that it would spread to the roof, and Hickman had tiles removed so that any danger could be observed. The women who occupied the rooms on the east side of the quadrangle were taken from them, and their furniture was later taken to the upper hall, to avoid damage from water. Because of the early hour, the fire was extinguished before many Guildford people were about. At 9 o'clock St John's Ambulance volunteers served tea, coffee, milk, Bovril and biscuits to the firemen and others, and also provided transport to take some of the residents to the homes of friends. Prayers in chapel were said as usual at 10 o'clock.

Gates's buildings were completely destroyed. Although the Three Pigeons was old, and mainly of wooden construction, fire damage was mostly to the roof and second floor; water did damage to the lower floors. Temporary covering was put onto the gaps in the hospital roof. Eight of the sisters lodged for a while out of the hospital, and the Governors allowed them an additional half crown a week for this time. A service of thanksgiving was held in the chapel on Sunday 2 July, and by 25 August all the rooms were back in occupation. The cost of repairs after the fire was met by an insurance claim of £288.2s.

The removal of adjacent buildings, some of which had been built right up to the hospital walls, made it possible for the outside of the property to be inspected more carefully.

The Reformed Community

The fire had not damaged the east window of the chapel, but it was seen that the stonework had decayed. In August 1916 the Governors decided to ask Harry Redfern, of Bedford Row London, to make a report on the windows. Redfern had been a pupil of Henry Woodyer, but some years after Woodyer's work at the hospital. There was some delay, and Redfern's recommendations were not received until early in 1918. It was decided to make a public appeal for the repair of the windows, and this brought in £339.18.2d. This made it possible to repair the north window as well. The glass was taken to London for repair and releading by Lowndes & Drury, at a cost of £140. The stonework was made good by Stanley Ellis, for £151.6.9d. Fees and other expenses amounted to £40.0.11d. A further £20 was spent in 1919 on the tracery of the east window.

Shortly after the fire, Palmer drew up a report on the conditions in which the residents lived, and presented it to the Governors in September 1916. He said that the brothers who did the portering were on duty for four months in the year, for fourteen hours a day. Their average age was 77, and they had to be out of doors in all weathers. The Governors told Palmer to rearrange the duties. He pointed out that rooms and staircases were decorated only when there was a vacancy. The rooms of long-lived residents were therefore in need of decoration. It was agreed that they might be done one by one. No action, however, was taken over the payments to the two nurses (17/9d and 13/9d) or the weekly distribution of eight shillings, even though the master urged that the purchasing power of money was reduced.

Palmer's care for the fabric continued. The Ascension day perambulation through Gates's property in 1917 led him to report a deterioration of the east wall after the fire, and that the foundations of the south-east chimney stack were exposed. He also noted that a timber and glass structure had been built against the hospital wall, and there was still much inflammable material there. Later in the year the Governors asked the architect T.R. Clemence[15] to make a survey. He reported that the chimney leaned two inches south and two and a half inches west, but there were no cracks. He also found that the north-west chimney leaned at least six inches, and should be strengthened. Repairs were done, costing £175. Only £100 had been set aside for this, and the balance was made up by not building an additional cowshed which the tenant of Rumbeams had asked for. A system of house visitors was adopted, two Governors regularly inspecting the hospital. They frequently found defects, but a serious consideration of the condition of the building was not given until 1920.

The hospital accounts for 1916 shewed a deficit of £20. On 22 March the Mayor, William Shawcross, as chairman of the Governors, made a statement. He accepted that some expenditure was urgent, to improve the sanitary provision on the women's side, to clean and renovate the residents' rooms, to point the east wall and to eliminate the overdraft of £500. He suggested that this could be done by reducing the payments to the Rector of Holy Trinity and to the medical officer, by stopping the garden contract and having the work done voluntarily by residents, and by economy in the use of gas. The Governors discussed the Mayor's suggestions, but took no definite action. Shawcross wrote to

Abbot's Hospital Guildford

insist that the coal allowance should be suspended, as allowed by the scheme, and said that he would raise a subscription for coal so that the residents should not suffer hardship. As his advice was not taken, Shawcross attended no further meetings. He reported the controversy to the Charity Commission, who asked for copies of the accounts for the three preceding years. In January 1918 the Governors considered a revolutionary suggestion from the Commission - that those residents who were eligible should apply for old age pensions, introduced by Asquith's government in 1909.[16] Those who were given pensions should have their hospital payments reduced, so saving money. The Governors replied that they did not wish to follow this course of action. Nonetheless, by the summer of 1920, all those entitled to a pension were receiving it, the sums ranging from two shillings to six shillings, and "several of the Inmates were truly grateful to receive this additional help". In that year an anonymous offer of £500 was made through Kirwan, to be invested for the increase of the residents' allowances. When it was perceived that this would have the effect of reducing their pensions, the offer seems to have been withdrawn, as the donor would not wish to relieve the state of its responsibilities.

Early in 1917 Palmer suggested that the garden should become more productive. He had been clearing shrubs and flowers away so that food could be grown. He asked that the gardener should concentrate on that, while the flower beds in the courtyard could be kept by himself, with the help of brothers. Later in the year he reported that this was working well, and it continued. In 1926 it was noted that the brothers and sisters usually had a weekly share of three varieties of vegetables.

The keeping of anniversaries became more popular as the twentieth century advanced, and it was decided to observe the tercentenary of the hospital's foundation. In May 1918 Kirwan wrote to the Archbishop of Canterbury on behalf of the Governors, inviting him to take part. Davidson replied that he was "sympathetically inclined and ready to co-operate". The celebration was held on 26 July 1919, beginning with the eucharist in the chapel at 10 o'clock. In the afternoon there was a procession from the hospital to Holy Trinity for a service, at which Archbishop Davidson preached on Psalm 145, verse 4, "One generation shall praise thy works unto another". A tea party in the common hall for the Archbishop, the Governors, the Corporation and the residents was paid for by the Mayor, W.S. Taverner, who had succeeded Shawcross.

In 1920 further thought for the condition of the building was given, and at the same time the insurance valuation was raised from £10,500 to £21,000, and the furniture owned by the Governors from £1000 to £2000. It was suggested that a thorough survey of the hospital should be commissioned. Nothing was done about this until 1923, after the master had reported, in August 1922, that ninety-nine of the windows needed attention, with work for a mason, an iron worker, a glazier and a painter. Redfern was invited to make the survey, and his fee of twenty guineas was approved. Redfern's report was passed on to T.R. Clemence, and his recommendations were followed. Repairs were started by Tribe & Robinson in May 1924, costing £394.10.7d. Clemence's fee was £15.

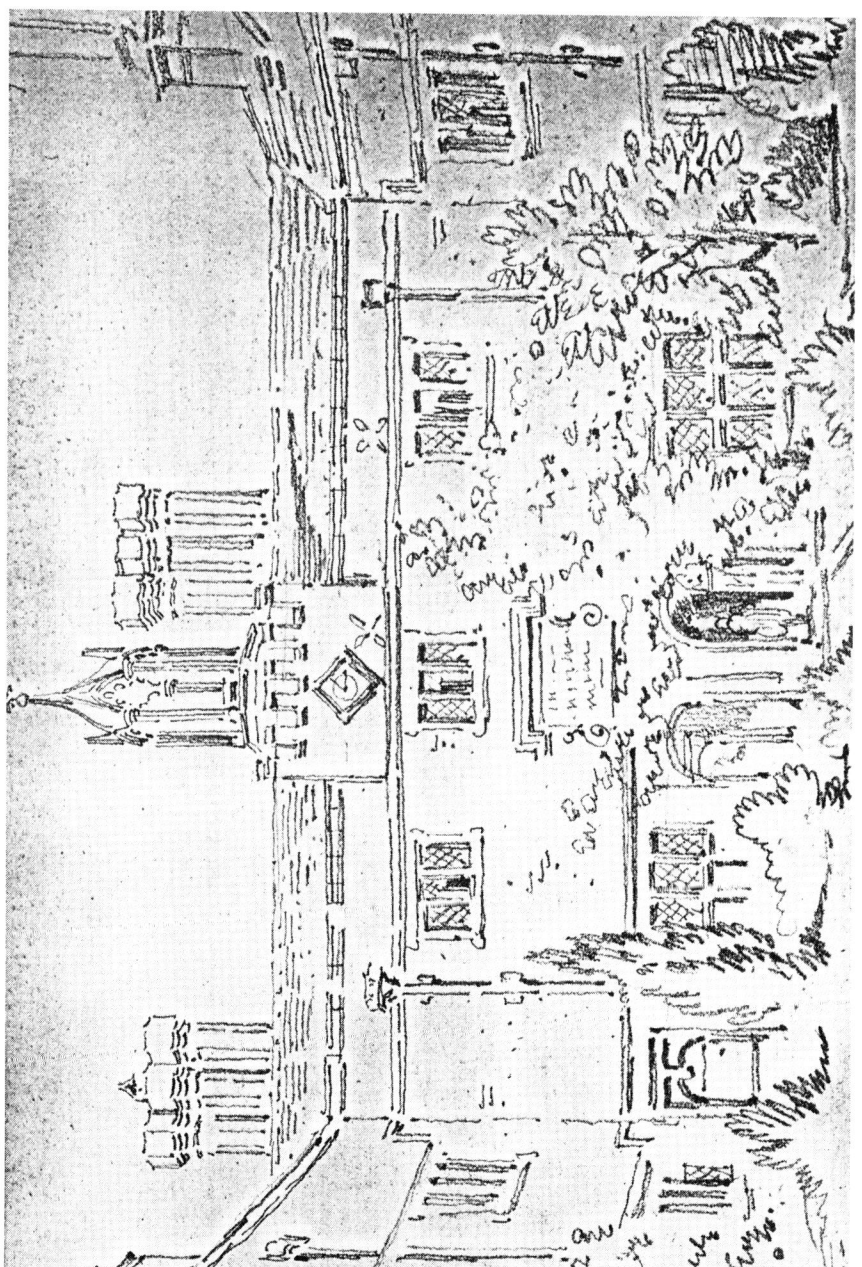

1. The courtyard in 1837

2. The House of Industry in 1822

3. The High Street front c1840

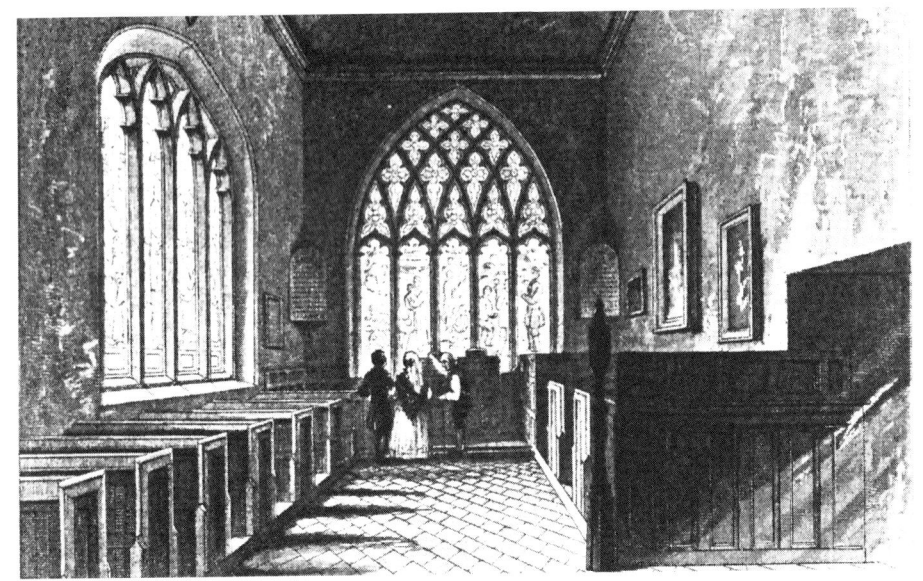

4. The chapel

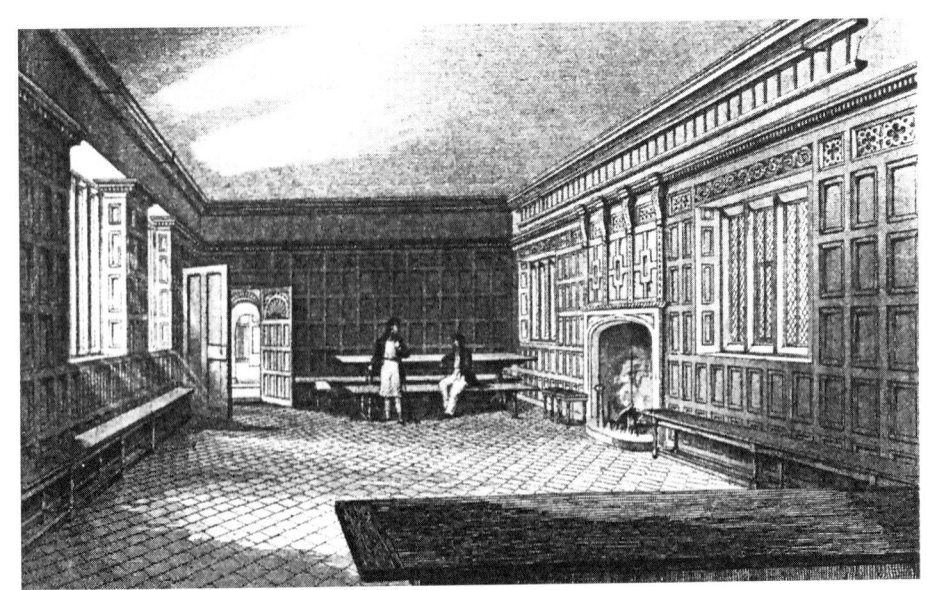

5. The hall

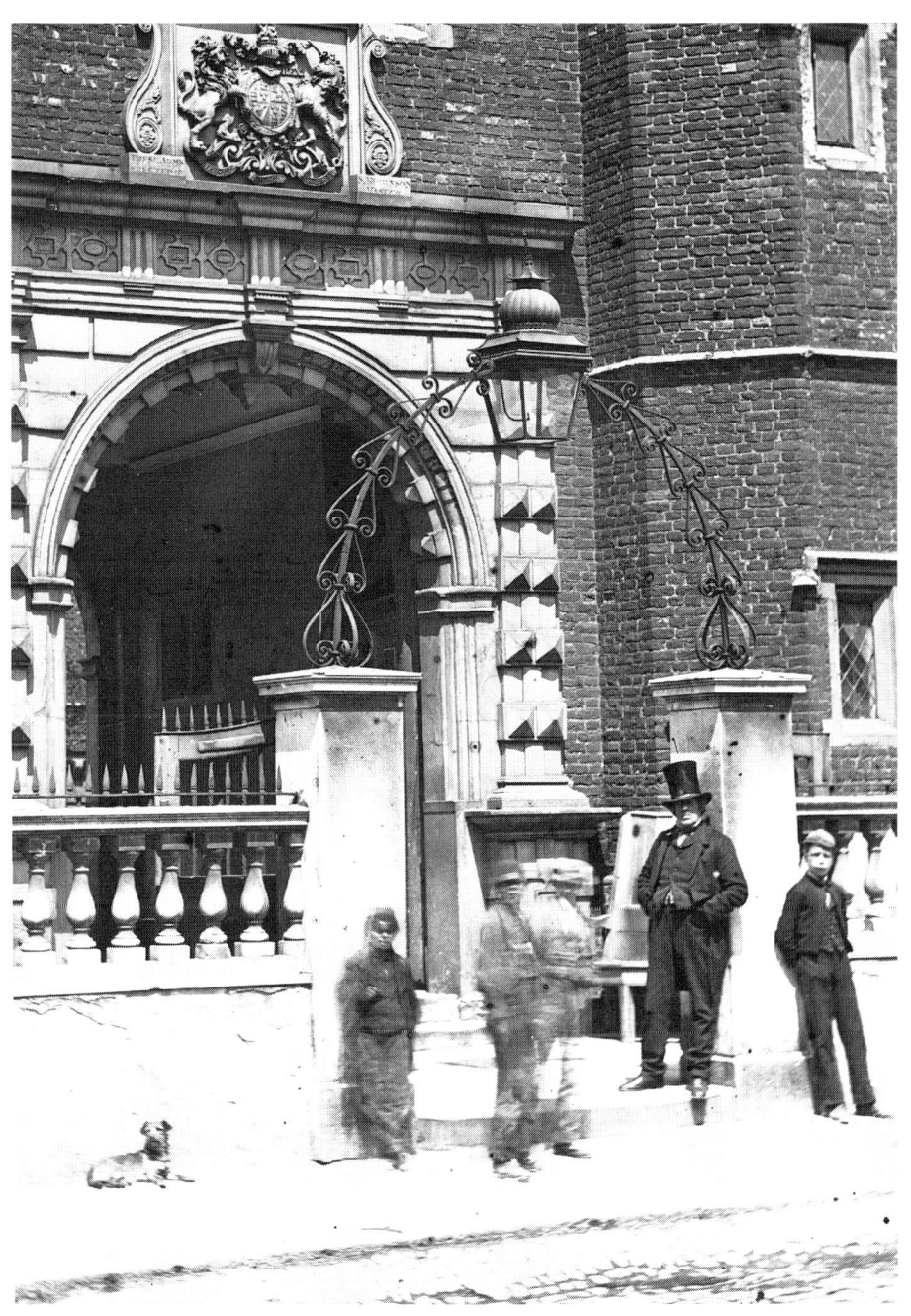
6. The Hospital Gateway c1865

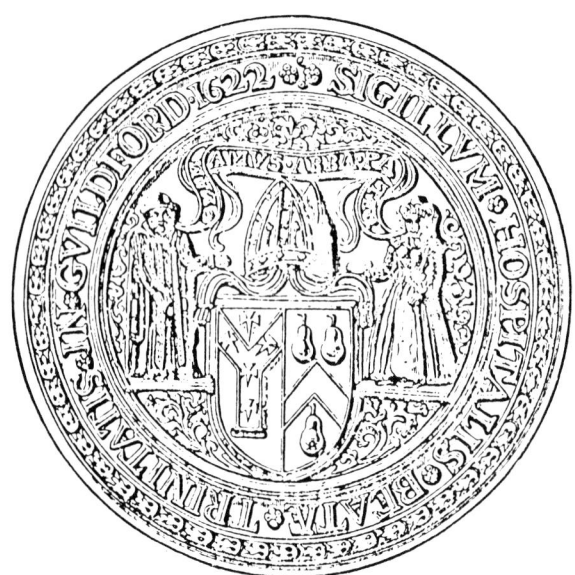

7. The Hospital seal

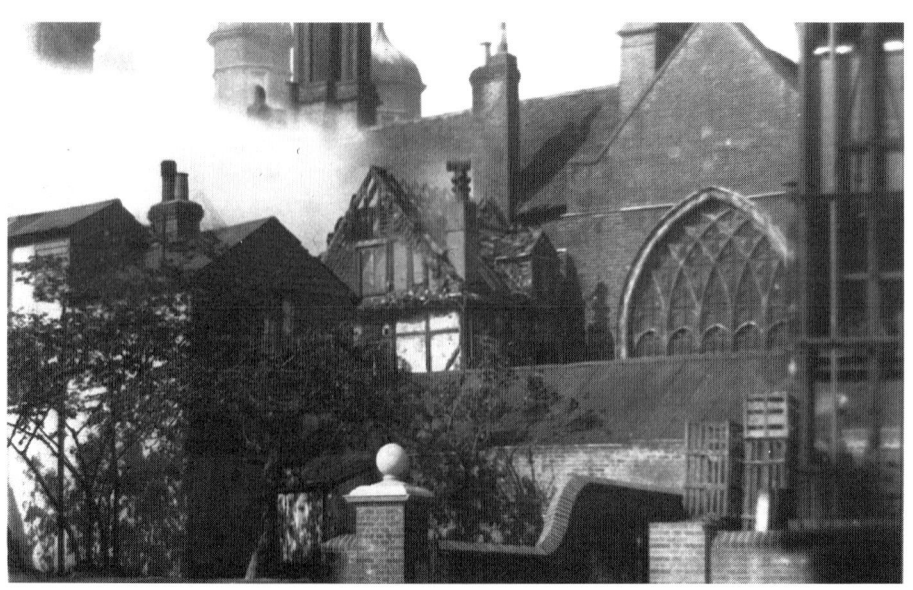

8. The fire of 1916

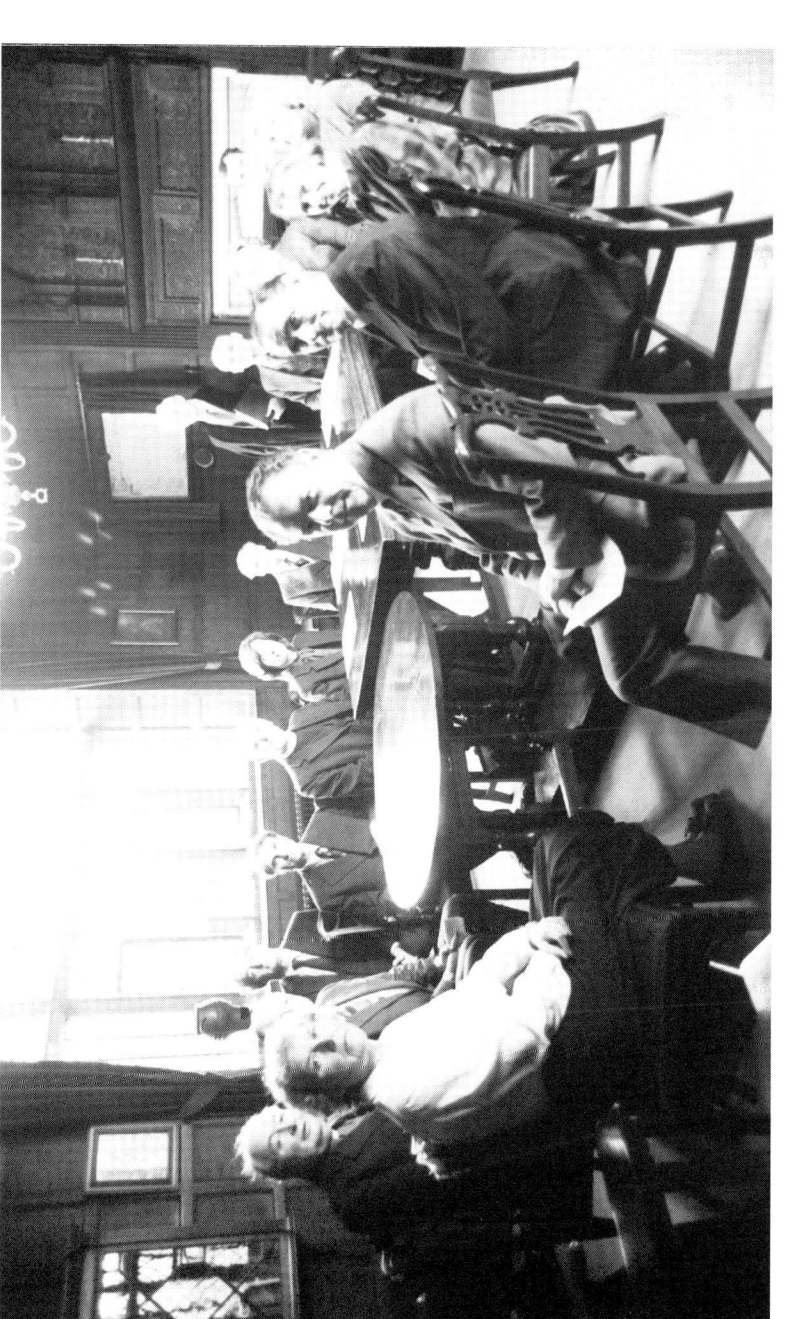

9. The Governors' meeting 1984

left to right: R.C.A. Carey, Mrs G.E. Pullan, C.J.K. Boyce, J. Daniel, R.G.K. Burgess, B. Taylor, Mrs F. Cox (Secretary), R.H. Percy (Clerk), B.T. Clarke, H.G. Taylor (Master), J.F. Brown, R.G.H. Beatrip, Mrs J.B. Golding, Mrs E.M. Cobbett, D.E. Weir-Rhodes, Mrs J. Baddeley

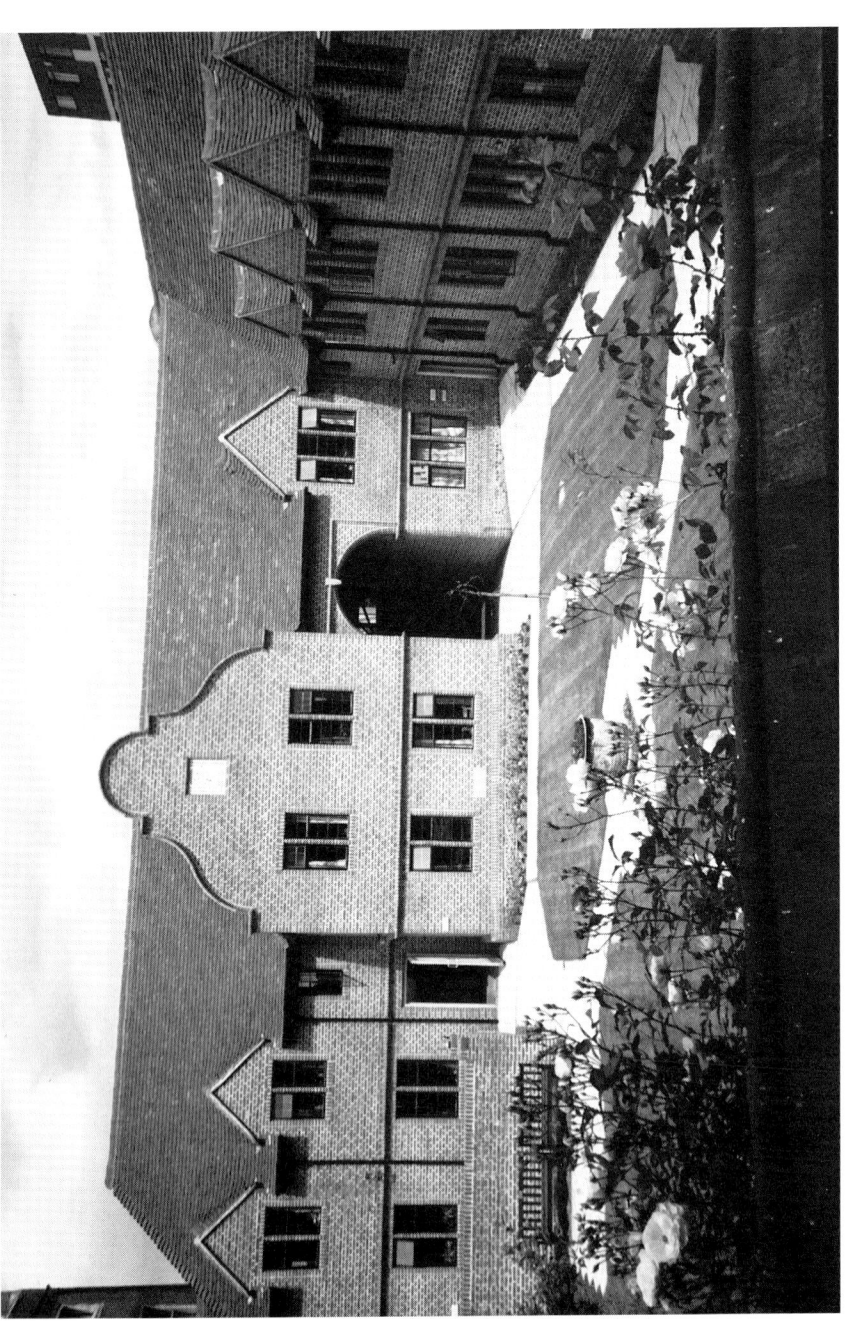

10. The new courtyard

The Reformed Community

In 1921 portering duties were again considered. The men took it in turn, and much time was taken up by the growing number of visitors. "The London 'Bus traffic has greatly increased the type of visitor whose aim is to saunter about, but shew no interest in,or knowledge of anything." The porter's room had for some time been used as a coal cellar. In 1922 it was considered whether the coal might be kept in the cellars below the north wing. The room of one of the brothers was also reduced in size to make a coal store. In 1924 the decision was made that coal should be stored in the cellar below the common hall. The distance that the cellar was from the old people's rooms was a subject of an anonymous letter received in 1925, most of which was a complaint about the "Lavatory accomadation", which was inadequate and remote. The Governors agreed to consider these matters, as they often did when suggestions or complaints were received.

The motor cars in the High Street made the crossing to church dangerous for the residents, and Palmer wondered whether special constables could be detailed to stop the traffic when necessary. Other changes came. Dr C.J. Sells resigned after forty-four years as medical officer, in 1923. He had succeeded his father in 1879. His successor was Dr G.M. Bluett. His annual payment was £22, out of which he was to provide medicine. Towards the end of Dr Sells's time, in 1922, the medical examination of applicants for hospital rooms began. The vice-master, James Williamson, died in 1925, aged 96, having served since 1906. He had been able to retain the office because another brother performed his duties.

By 1923 gowns were worn only in chapel and by the porter on duty. A new design had been adopted in 1914, found "much more comfortable and easy to wear than the old ones". These had been washed and patched and altered, and handed on from one person to another, and new ones were needed.

During the years that Palmer was master, the Governors disposed of much of their estates, including most of the remaining farms of the original endowment. The Charity Commission's approval had always to be obtained, for the sale and for the price, and the Governors had to invest the proceeds, to maintain or increase the endowment income. In 1913 approval was given for the sale of a quarter of an acre at Merrow for £100, for the enlargement of the churchyard. The money realised bought £132.17.7d consols. In 1916 the Governors were permitted to pay for improvements at Highlands farm at Horsham. Stock nominally worth £1205.3.10d was sold for £799.17.3d to pay for the new cowsheds. This money was to be reinvested within fifteen years.

In June 1920 the Governors obtained a new valuation of the farms for insurance - £11,185, an increase of £4460. This was for Highlands and Hornbrook at Horsham, Hall Place at Merrow, Shepherd's at Stoughton and Rumbeams at Ewhurst. Two months later the tenant at Rumbeams offered to buy it for £2000. The Governors spoke of £4000, and in October asked for £3000. The Charity Commission did not approve of the sale of land during the term of a lease, but because a strong request had been made, they would permit the sale, after public notice, if no objection was made. The farm was sold early

Abbot's Hospital Guildford

in 1922, and the proceeds, £1808, were invested in £1919.18.7d 5% war stock. The annual income would be £95.19s, nearly double the rent from the farm.

In 1923 permission was received to sell a strip of land in Trodds Lane Merrow for road widening, for £100. In this case the price received in 1924 was higher, £150, used to buy £146.5.4d 5% war stock. In 1925 Send meadow was sold for £130, invested in £134.3s $3^{1}/_{2}$% war stock.

In November 1923 the Mayor, J.B. Rapkins, reaching the end of his first year of service, reported that he had inspected the hospital lands, and recommended that both Shepherd's farm and Hall Place should be sold for building development when it became possible. Part of Shepherd's farm was sold in 1926, but not for housing. The Borough Council already rented four acres as allotments. The Governors were prepared to sell them to the Council for £2800, and another seventeen acres for £3500, to become a recreation ground. The Ministry of Health considered that the price was too high, and the Charity Commission approved the sale for £6000, with which £7946.10.4d $3^{1}/_{2}$% conversion stock was bought.

At Merrow there was an exchange of part of the Hall Place land in 1926. The Governors acquired a piece that was more suitable for development, and £500 as well. This (less £44.10s expenses) was invested in £611.17.1d $3^{1}/_{2}$% conversion stock. Before the exchange was completed, W.A.C. Burling offered to buy the whole estate for £10,500. The farm was advertised, and was sold at the end of the year for £13,000, half of which was invested in £8490.17.4d $3^{1}/_{2}$% conversion stock, and half in £7655.17.2d 4% consols.

Palmer's genial mastership was generally appreciated. In 1921 the Mayor, G.W. Franks, suggested that the master should be rewarded (at the expense of the residents) with a 10% share of the money in the visitors' boxes. Palmer declined this offer twice, but he did accept a gratuity of five guineas from hospital funds. For the whole of 1926 the Master was in poor health. In November E.C. Kirwan, the Rector of Holy Trinity, thinking ahead, raised the question of the possibility of a married master. This was left for consideration. Within a month, Philip Palmer died, on 13 December. His funeral at Holy Trinity was three days later.

A committee was formed on 1 December 1926 to consider the appointment of a new master. The approval of the Archbishop of Canterbury and of the Charity Commission was obtained for increasing the salary to £100, and the position was advertised for three weeks, early in 1927. There was only one applicant, and he was not considered suitable. Kirwan was asked to approach the Charity Commission to seek approval for changes in the nature of the appointment. He explained that the advertisement had been unsuccessful, and asked for a further increase of the salary, to £150, possible because of the hospital's improved income. He also asked for permission to appoint a married man. The Commissioners' reply, dated 9 March, allowed the larger salary. With regard to a married master it was pointed out that the master was one of those whom the charity was designed

The Reformed Community

to benefit. An alteration could be made only by Parliament. The Commission would prepare a scheme if it was certain that there would be no opposition, so that a bill could be introduced in 1928. In the meanwhile the Governors should advertise again for a single man.

On 6 April 1927 the Governors considered three applications, and decided to interview Ernest George Reignolds Wale, a bachelor aged fifty-seven. Wale appeared before the board on 9 April, and he was appointed. The following day he was taken to the chapel to meet the brothers and sisters. The Archbishop's approval was given on 1 June.[17] The master's lodging was wired for electricity, as a cost of £12.6.6d, and Wale's long occupation of it began. He had first come to Guildford in 1890, to work in a bookshop. Later he bad been a bank official in London. Like Palmer he was a keen churchman, well known in anglo-catholic circles. For forty-eight years he was secretary general of the Guild of Servants of the Sanctuary.

The Governors continued to consider how the hospital could be made more convenient and suitable for modern life. In July 1927 it was decided to discuss this with Clemence. Lavatories were once again included, and the possibility of providing baths was suggested, as well as "quarters for a Porter and Portress". Clemence agreed that there should be a consultant, as structural alterations might be necessary, and the noted architect and writer Walter Hindes Godfrey was secured. Clemence produced drawings for a scheme that would give a bathroom and lavatory for each set of four rooms, lit by skylights behind the parapets. The staircases would need to be altered to make this possible. The master's lodgings would also be given a bathroom. For the nurses three rooms would be altered to provide bedrooms and a bathroom and lavatory. Drinking water would also be laid on to the staircases. He did not make plans for the porter's accommodation, but considered that the rooms leading from the gateway would be sufficient. An improvements committee was formed, to consider the architect's proposals.

Objections were raised to altering the staircases, and the alternative was suggested that the lavatories and bathrooms should be made in the basements. These were really cellars, and while those on the west side had stairs, those on the east could be reached only by ladders. Godfrey favoured this scheme, and Clemence came to support it too, but the Governors did not, as it would be very inconvenient for the residents, especially those with upstairs rooms. Later in 1928 it was said that while the master and the nurses should have baths, the residents should not, as they were too old to use them. Slipper baths and a supply of hot and cold water would be sufficient. Clemence's proposals were submitted to the Charity Commission. Early in 1929 the Commissioners replied that they approved the idea of lavatories and baths, but not of altering the staircases. They suggested a new building for them. They also regretted the reduction by two of the number of residents that the alterations would entail. They also asked that the opinion of the eminent architect William Douglas Caroë should be obtained. Caroë favoured the basement proposals, but the Governors persevered with the staircase plan, and that gained the Charity Commission's approval, in August 1929. Tenders were invited, but there

Abbot's Hospital Guildford

was a further delay. While examining the building to assess the proposals, Caroë noticed that there was damage by death watch beetle. Clemence was instructed to examine the whole hospital, and it was found that much needed to be done. In 1929 £950.7.6d had already been spent (rebuilding three chimneys, repairs to leadwork, garden walls and steps, and general repairs and painting), so it was decided that the improvements must be put off while the infected woodwork was made good, and other necessary work completed. This phase of restoration was carried out by R. Wood and Son, and came to an end in 1930, at the cost of £3173.10.1d. Clemence said that more was needed, but the Governors decided to turn to improvement. While the north-east hospital wall was being underpinned, in connexion with new building by Cow and Gate, the foundation stone was discovered below ground level. In 1931 it was inserted in the wall of the chapel, behind the altar.

In March 1931 the Governors decided to delay the improvements no longer. The master was to be provided with a bathroom and lavatory on the ground floor. Quarters for the porter were to comprise living room and bedroom, with bathroom and lavatory, and the nurses were to have similar accommodation. In the east and west wings each staircase was to have a sink half way up the stairs, and a lavatory at a higher level. Similar provision was to be made for the other rooms occupied by residents. Water would be laid on, and electric lights installed. In order to make the rearrangements possible, the Charity Commission gave temporary permission for the number of brothers to be reduced by two. This work was to be paid for out of the hospital's improved income.

The contract was given to H.W. Frampton & Co., and work began on 1 June. By September the lavatories and sinks on the women's side were complete, to the great satisfaction of the sisters. While this was being done, further infesting by death watch beetle was found. The women were sent out into lodgings while this was remedied. Brickwork replaced some timber and plaster partitions, and remaining woodwork was treated with Kenford Fluid. It was decided that the heating of the hall and chapel should be separate from the supply of hot water for the baths and sinks. Frampton's work cost £2020.2.lld, £183.2.1ld more than the estimate because of the eradication of the beetle. Carling, Gill & Carling were paid £61 for the water heating appliances. Fees paid to Clemence were £146.18.6d, and to Caroë six guineas.

It was also discovered that the roof of the muniment room in the gatehouse was badly infested. Unsound timber was renewed, and the principal beam was replaced with a rolled steel joist. At the same time a strong-room was formed in the southwest turret, costing £58.17.6d. The total cost of this gatehouse work, done by Higlett & Hammond, was £733.8s, with fees to Clemence of £34.3.4d. In 1933 repairs to the hospital roof were found to be necessary. The north slope of the east wing, the south block and the south-west corner were stripped and rebattened. This contract was given to G.W. Franks, and was begun on 8 June, to cost within £350.

The gardens were expensive to maintain, and Wale did not share Palmer's enthusiasm. In 1932 the flower beds in the courtyard were removed and relaced with lawns - a change

The Reformed Community

which won general approval. In 1933 it was realised that the cost of cultivating the lower garden, £28.14s, was more than three times the value of vegetables produced, estimated at £8.18s. It was decided to put the garden down to grass, and to buy vegetables for the residents. Mowing was expected to cost £6.12s, and the expense of providing vegetables was precisely forecast, £19.19.11d. Modern circumstances thus brought to an end one of the founder's arrangements for the welfare of the brothers and sisters.

In 1934 a representative of the Midland Clock Company of Derby inspected the clock, and reported that it was clogged with unsuitable grease. Two years later it was dismantled, and cleaned by Johnsons of Croydon. The paving of the entrance to the hospital was improved, and the gas light was replaced with electricity, the fitting being retained as an early example of a gas lamp. When rooms were decorated the old fireplaces, which had been made smaller in 1713-21, were restored to their original size and appearance. These were early examples in the hospital of consideration of design and historical interest, rather than concern simply for utility.

The years before the second world war saw some special events. The three hundredth anniversary of the founder's death was observed on 4 August 1933 in a sombre way. The curate of Holy Trinity, H.D. Pilcher, celebrated the eucharist, and the flag was flown at half mast. A wreath, provided by the Mayor, was displayed on an easel in the gateway, and later placed on the Archbishop's tomb. The silver jubilee of King George V fell on 6 May 1935. It was proposed that the residents should be given double pay that week, but this was defeated. Instead they were given a day out, and by their request it was to Portsmouth. The cost was £8.4.6d. The Archbishop of Canterbury, C.G. Lang, agreed to make a private visit to the hospital on 13 July 1933. Because of a meeting of the committee dealing with the White Paper on India the visit could not take place then. Instead he came on 21 July 1935, and planted the yew tree. In 1937 the coronation of King George VI and Queen Elizabeth was celebrated with a motor trip to Southsea, in which the ladies of the Caleb Lovejoy Foundation were invited to join.

In 1932 the question of providing meals for the residents was raised again. There had been a gas stove in the kitchen since about 1919 for those who wished to use it, but Wale considered that many minor ailments were caused by badly cooked food, especially among the inexpert men. He suggested charging two shillings a week for seven midday meals. The sum collected, £104, would cover much of the cost of the food and the wages of the cook. The committee was asked to discuss this with the medical officer, but no action was taken.

No gaudies had been held for several years, but a tea party was always held after Christmas. On 8 January 1936 this was expanded by a tree, with presents. Another additional treat was provided by Miss Edith Ide of Johannesburg, a descendant of the Abbot family. For several years she sent money for a tea party. In 1935 she visited the hospital, and presided over the party herself. In 1932 the brothers and sisters asked for the closing time for the gates to be 9 o'clock in the winter instead of 8. This was cautiously agreed to. In 1936

Abbot's Hospital Guildford

it was decided that the gates should remain open until 10 o'clock from May to September, to take advantage of British Summer Time.

In 1934 it was estimated that each resident cost the hospital twelve shillings and eightpence a week (coal 2s, elecricity and gas 1s, vegetables 4d, medicines 8d, share of gift boxes 8d, weekly allowance 8s). All save one received the ten shillings old age pension. The exception was given an allowance equal to the pension until eligible for it.

It generally appears to have been a contented community. In 1937 the Governors were told that a new brother, J. Pyke, had written to say that he was "as happy as a sparrow in a wheatfield and very comfortable - everybody kind and sympathetic. That is as near to Paradise as humanity is likely to get in this world." His letter was accompanied by eight doyleys for the Governors, with a promise of four more.

In 1933 the medical officer, Dr Bluett, asked for an increase in his remuneration after ten years' service. It was raised from £22 to £30. In 1937 Dr Bluett retired, and was replaced by Dr G.H. Peake, who had often acted as deputy. In 1938 Dr Peake retired, and was succeeded by Dr H.P. Gabb.

The allowances for the clerk and chaplain were revised in 1934, and it was agreed that the clerk's payment should be doubled to £80, and that the hospital should pay for stationery, postage and typing. This was approved by the Charity Commission. The Commission did not, however, approve the proposal to increase the chaplain's remuneration from £10 to £20. The ruling of 1869 was repeated, that the office of chaplain was not provided for by the scheme of management; the hospital was not an ecclesiastical charity, and the beneficiaries need not be members of the Church of England; the Rector had no duties "beyond giving such spiritual assistance to those Almspeople who required his help" - and they were, in any case, all his parishioners. Furthermore, as a Governor, Kirwan should never have been appointed. However, in view of his long service no objection would be raised - but he must be paid no more than £10. The Governors were astonished by this ruling; they had always assumed that it was a Church institution, and considered applying for a new scheme, but decided against hasty action. E.C. Kirwan died on 15 December 1936. The Reverend H.D. Pilcher, curate at Holy Trinity, now the Cathedral, who had acted since November, was appointed chaplain in May 1937. He was to be paid £10, while the new Provost, E.G. Southam, was to receive the statutory thirty shillings. Pilcher left to be Rector of Holmbury St Mary in 1938. The Bishop of Guildford, J.V. Macmillan, and Southam suggested that a retired priest, G.M. Hutton, should be appointed, and this was confirmed in May.

Although rooms were prepared for a porter it was decided in 1932 not to appoint to the post, as one of the brothers was looking after the boilers for five shillings a week, and willing to continue. In the following year the rooms were designated for the vice-master when a new appointment was needed. The brothers continued to take turns for portering duties, and a light-weight cloak was bought for use in the summer. The vice-master, J. Buck, died on 19 July 1938, having been elected to the hospital in 1910 especially to hold that office. No-one in the hospital was thought suitable to be chosen to follow him, and the Governors considered advertising in the local newspapers, and paying the vice-master £20 a year instead of one pound a quarter, if the Charity Commission approved. The matter rested there until the unexpected meeting on 8 December.

Requests were received in 1930 for the purchase of the rest of Shepherd's Farm for £9000, for £10,500 from the tenant, and for £11,250. These were declined. Then the Borough Council offered £12,000. "The land is required for the building of houses which are so urgently needed in the Borough." The Charity Commission was consulted, and approval was given. The Council's offer was increased to £12,500, but Charles Osenton and Company, Estate Agents, outbid the Borough, and bought the land for £13,000. This was invested in £13,977.16.4d 4% consols. The Council had already bought a strip of land for road widening earlier in 1930, for £300, invested in £383.19.7d 3% conversion stock, and a further small piece for £10 in 1931, invested in £13.9.4d 3½% conversion stock.

Negotiations began in 1931 for the sale of two plots of land at Merrow, amounting to 20.98 acres, for housing development. The valuation was £250 an acre, but the purchaser wished to reduce the price to £4000 because of restrictions on use imposed by the Rural District Council. The reduction was refused, and the sale was concluded in 1932. The proceeds, £5250, were invested in £5225.6.6d 3½% conversion stock. More land was sold at Merrow to the Surrey County Council in 1933, and the price, £112.10s, was used to purchase £11.9s 3½% conversion stock. In 1935 there was an offer to buy Hornbrook Farm for £2000. The Governors declined because it was not available for sale at that time. Highlands Farm was frequently discussed by the Governors, because of outstanding rent, and requests for repairs and alterations. In 1936 it was decided to build two additional cottages there, at the estimated cost of £900. The Charity Commission's approval was received early in 1937. The cost rose to £1178.8s because of soil drainage. These cottages were paid for from hospital income, which had improved because of the investment policy. In addition, in 1937, £1000 surplus was invested in £1017.1.3d local 3% loans.

On 31 December 1936 there was a chimney fire at 22 High Street, immediately to the west of the hospital, and attics were filled with smoke. There was continuing anxiety from fire risk because of the boxes and straw which the tenant, Arthur Grove, kept in the yard. In 1935 the Governors had begun to consider purchasing number 22, both to have control over it, and to enjoy rent from it. The owners, the executors of the Triggs Turner estate, were not then wishing to sell the property, but said that if circumstances changed they would give the first option to the tenant and the second to the hospital.

As recorded in chapter 3, the Governors of the hospital bought the Old Cloth Hall from the trustees of the Archbishop Abbot's Exhibition Foundation in 1934 for £4000, with expenses of the purchase amounting to £148.6.1d. The Charity Commission approved of the purchase, and suggested that the price should be found from the sale of conversion stock. Clark's College Limited had occupied the building since 1933, and continued to

Abbot's Hospital Guildford

use it as a school. The charge for using the yard as a playground was raised from £1 to £4.

Archbishop Abbot's School had used the hospital stable since 1929, but Clark's did not need it. It was leased to Arthur Grove for three years, for the yearly payment of £15.[18] In 1937 there was a long waiting list for hospital places, and the Governors decided that accommodation could be increased by adapting the stable to make a cottage for the nurses. Grove was given notice for his use of the building to end. T.R. Clemence produced plans in 1938, for a sitting room, with kitchen and larder on the ground floor, and two bedrooms, bathroom and lavatory upstairs, the expected cost being between £250 and £300. The estimates received were for £498, £515 and £542. Clemence was asked to find ways of bringing the price down. This was done with the advice of the London architect Herbert Passmore. The work was given to Stanley Ellis Ltd, and the cost was eventually £412.6.7d.

The proposal to convert the stable into a cottage was submitted to the Charity Commission, who sent the Assistant Commissioner, Leonard F. Ford to visit the hospital, and interview the Governors at a special meeting on 8 December 1938. The visit was virtually an inspection. Ford looked at the stable to see what the Governors wanted to do, and also the chapel, hall, kitchen, two of the residents' rooms, a lavatory and the garden. He discussed with the Governors the composition of the Board, and its chairmanship, the investment of surplus funds, the vice-mastership and the appointment of porter. A second special meeting was held on 22 February 1939 to consider the Charity Commission's recommendations.

1. An extraordinary repair fund of £10,000 should be built up, begun with £3722.4.6d local 3% loans and their accumulated income, and increased annually by £200 from the Governors' investment income. This was agreed to.

2. The conversion of the stable into a cottage was approved.

3. While the removal of the nurses to the cottage would leave two rooms for additional residents, the proportion of twelve brothers to eight sisters should not be altered unless there were no male applicants or no suitable ones.

4. Two nurses for twenty-two brothers and sisters was more than necessary, but it would be permitted if the assistant helped to look after the older residents and cleaned the cottage. The Governors decided that in future the assistant nurse should be called the nurse's assistant.

5. It was recommended that the residents' income should be made up to twenty shillings a week (including pension). That, with free housing, light, heat and nursing "should be enough to enable the inmates to live in reasonable comfort". The Governors agreed, but allowed the extra two shillings only to future residents; but later they rescinded this decision, and no increase was made at all.

6. The medical officer's salary was to be not more than £40, a permitted rise from £30.

The Reformed Community

7. Approval was given to the appointment of a porter, who would do the work of gardener, stoker, casual labourer and cleaner. The proposed payment was to be submitted to the Commission. The clerk estimated the 1938 cost of this work to be £67.17.6d. The Governors recommended allowing a wage of £2.5s, with free use of rooms, and coal and light. The master was to draw up a list of duties. The Provost, who had been using the porter's room as an office, was asked to leave it.

8. The Governors' proposal to advertise for a paid vice-master was not approved. The Commissioners considered that "brothers should be appointed in order of application, other things being equal". The Governors accepted this, and in May 1939 elected the senior brother, G.S.Wilson.

9. A change in the composition of the governing body would need an Act of Parliament. The Governors decided not to press for this.

In April the master reported that the nurse, Miss C.E. Duncan, was anxious to occupy the porter's lodge. This was allowed, and it was settled that the cottage should be the house for the porter. The Charity Commission agreed, and an advertisement was placed for a porter, whose wife should be the nurse's assistant, for a joint wage of £2.10s, with the cottage and free heat and light. Mr and Mrs E. Button were appointed from 11 December 1939.

The approach of war was discussed by the Governors in 1938, when the fear of attack from the air was rising. In July it was decided that the cellar under the hall should be cleaned, and electric light laid on, so that it could be "used as a refuge for the Inmates". The porter's lodge was to become an air raid warden's post. In July the Governors resolved to purchase one stirrup pump, in case of fire from enemy action. When war was declared, the medical officer, Dr Gabb, was quickly called up; Dr D.Whittaker acted in his place. To prepare for the blackout, 26¼ yards of ARP black cloth were supplied by the Complete Art Furnisher, for £1.19.4d. The curtains were made up by M. Avery & Sons for £37.16.2d.

Despite worsening conditions - or perhaps to act while it was still possible, some improvements were made. In 1939 the Mayor, R.H. Tribe, and Lawrence Powell were asked to arrange for four new English oak doors for the entrances to the brothers' and sisters' staircases. They were made by A.H. Billimore & Son, and were in place by the end of the year, costing £40.18s. Billimore also redecorated the chapel, for £17.10s. Clemence was asked to alter the bathroom to which sisters had access, dividing it into two, and putting in a second bath. This was done for £70.10s by Higlett & Hammond Ltd.

Archbishop Abbot's tomb was still regarded as the responsibility of the hospital. In January 1938 the Governors discussed a report by the architect W.H.R. Blacking and Miss Janet Becker, whose restoration of old paintwork was regarded by some as controversial. Her advice was taken and she started work in July. The cost was £43.2.6d, with £2.8.6d for her report. The 1889 iron railings were taken away to see whether the appearance without them would be preferred.[19] Three days after the declaration of war, Southwell asked whether the effigy should be put into a place of safety. The other Governors "considered that the Tomb was quite as safe in the Church as it would be if placed elsewhere", but instructed the clerk to find out what the Governors of the Croydon hospital were proposing to do with Archbishop Whitgift's tomb in the Parish Church there. They replied that they were doing nothing, so the Guildford Governors left the security of Abbot's tomb to the church wardens. They did decide to protect the north window of the chapel, and it was boarded up.

The first winter of the war was very cold, and there was a shortage of fuel. The hall and the chapel were not heated, and morning prayers were suspended. One of the sisters asked if "her wireless set might be attached to the electric current". The Governors consulted the borough electrical engineer, and then decided to refuse the request. Later in 1940 the request was renewed, and approval was given, the cost of electrical points being sixteen shillings for each room. The house committee and the master were to frame rules for the use of the wirelesses. The following year one of the sets burst into flames, but no damage was done to the room or the brother. Residents were warned to turn their instruments off in thundery weather, and they were to be examined quarterly. In 1942 it was discovered that some residents were dangerously plugging electric rings into their wireless points. This was prohibited. Later in 1942 it was discovered that at least two residents had sought wartime comfort in keeping cats. The ban on pets was to be enforced.

The Governors voted in 1940 to increase the master's payment from £150 to £200. The Charity Commission refused to allow this, on the grounds that there had been "no appreciable rise in the cost of living" since 1927 when the salary had been fixed. Permission was given for a £25 rise in 1941. In 1940 the porter was given a weekly cost of living bonus of half a crown, increased to fifteen shillings in 1943.

In 1943 G.M. Hutton retired from the chaplaincy. He was replaced by the Reverend A.L. Gardiner, a retired priest who had come to live in Guildford. Later in 1943 the clerk, Frederick Elsley died. R.H. Percy was appointed on a temporary basis, to be considered for permanent engagement after the war. While he was away on active service his duties were carried out by Stewart Higgins of Smallpeice and Merriman.

The master suggested in 1940 that valuable furniture and pictures in the boardroom should be stored in a place of safety, and in March 1941 some chosen pieces were put into the cellar. That year the lawns in the lower garden were dug up so that vegetables could be grown there again. In September it was reported that nearly a ton of potatoes had been lifted.

The hospital was much affected by civil defence activities. The porter went through "a theoretical & practical Air Raid Warden's course". He asked for a ring in the refuge room for making tea; it would cost 14/6d. In 1940 it was agreed that planks should be laid on the rafters, to make movement easier for dealing with incendiary bombs, but this seems not to have been done until 1943. In November 1940 the Chief Constable asked for the use of the tower for an observation post "in connection with incendiary bombs, illicit lights etc." A small shed would be needed for the observers, "with a table and a Map and direction finding apparatus". The Governors agreed to this. The Home Office did not think that this was suitable, but the spotters' shed was erected, and Wale joined a committee to arrange a roster of watches, the headquarters being at the Three Pigeons. The Borough Council supplied sandbags in February 1941.

In 1943 it was reported that some residents had become careless about shewing lights during the blackout, especially in the early morning. The Governors warned that they would be liable to any penalties brought on them by this. Later that year the National Fire Service sent word that the hospital was on its priority list for attention if there was need. Advice was given on fire precaution and access to the roofs, and buckets of sand and water were put in readiness. Later in the year four more stirrup pumps were lent to the hospital, and pails of water put beside them. Most noticeable of all were three static water tanks put into the courtyard by the NFS in August 1944.

As the war drew to an end the hut on the gatehouse went out of use, and was removed in February 1945. The furniture and pictures were returned to the boardroom, and the north window of the chapel was uncovered. The static water tanks were removed in August. On Ascension Day, 10 May, the walking of the hospital bounds was resumed.

During these years the Governors were much concerned by the neighbouring property, 22 High Street. In 1940 the wartime awareness of fire risk directed attention to the inflammable material kept there, but requests to Arthur Grove, the insurance company and the owners had little effect. In December 1941 the Governors asked the trustees of the Triggs Turner estate if they would sell the property, and the consent of the Charity Commission for the purchase was obtained. A survey shewed that the High Street frontage was 12 feet, and the length along Jeffries Passage about 110 feet. The building had three floors, including a shop of 50 feet. The trustees asked for £5500, but the Charity Commission did not allow more than £5000. £4500 was raised by selling conversion stock, and the balance was found from income, as well as £140 for costs. The transaction was completed in 1942.

Grove's lease had expired in 1941. A new lease was negotiated for seven years from 23 September 1943, at £300 *per annum*, and a £275 deposit was claimed for repairs. The wireless and electrical business continued, A. Grove (Guildford) Limited, and the danger from fire risk was not lessened, and was commented on by the NFS.

The sale of Hornbrook farm was discussed in June 1944. It was then discovered that the tenant had built a bungalow on it. He agreed to be bought out of it for £990, which would include the fittings of the farm. The farm was sold by auction for £4050. After fees, charges and the compensation for the tenant had been settled, the Governors received £2785.14.3d, with which £2628.1.7d 3½% conversion stock was bought.

Abbot's Hospital Guildford

Soon after the end of the war, R.H. Percy returned from active service, and was confirmed in the post of clerk, which he held for many years. The residents shared the hardness of the times, and the hospital was glad to receive gifts on their behalf, men's shirts, pyjamas and underwear from a nursing home, rubber hot water bottles and grey blankets from the WVS.

In September 1945 the decision was taken to sell Highlands farm, the last of the original endowment properties. The Charity Commission permitted the sale for £11,000. After expenses had been paid, and £900 compensation given to the tenant on a valuation for stock, the Governors were able to invest £9609.2.4d in £9440.9.2d 3% savings bonds.

In 1947 the Charity Commission agreed that the weekly payment to the brothers and sisters might be raised, but not to more than twelve shillings. This was back-dated to 1 January. In 1948 approval was given for the master's salary to be increased from £175 to £210, and his fuel might be provided. In 1948 the running of the hospital cost £2702.1.7d, as this summary of the accounts shews.

property maintenance

rates	76.	13.	4
heating and lighting	220.	14.	9
repairs and replacements	163.	10.	6
insurance and tithe	97.	19.	4
cleaning	25.	0.	7
garden	5.	16.	0

payments for residents

pay	776.	7.	4
coal	192.	12.	2
clothing		10.	0
medicine	19.	15.	7

salaries

master	210.	0.	0
chaplain	20.	0.	0
medical officer	30.	0.	0
clerk	125.	0.	0
nurses	175.	17.	6
porter	229.	15.	0
vice-master	3.	0.	0
National Health Insurance	43.	1.	9
Employer's Liability Insurance	1.	14.	8

The Reformed Community

general expenses
professional charges	4.	4.	0
office expenses	63.	2.	7
sundries	17.	6.	6

provision for repairs
transfer to special fund	200.	0.	0

The income to support this expenditure was more than provided by investments, £2834.9s. In addition the hospital received

rents
for the Old Cloth Hall	179.	0.	0
for 22 High Street, with insurance	336.	8.	0
easements		2.	0
West Wantley farm annuity	12.	10.	0

miscellaneous
sale of guidebooks	28.	15.	0
sundry receipts		10.	0
	£557.	5.	0d

The total income was thus £3391.14s, leaving a balance of £689.12.5d

The use of electricity increased. In 1946 £6.18.10d was spent extending lighting to the master's kitchen and bathroom. In 1948 13 amp sockets were put into twenty-two rooms. Electric rings on brackets were supplied, the estimated cost of this being £250. A little later a fire alarm system was installed by H.P. Nott Ltd, costing £310.

On 10 June 1948 the Archbishop of Canterbury, G.F. Fisher, visited the hospital informally. He met the brothers and sisters in the guest chamber, and some of the Governors in the boardroom.

The architect, T.R. Clemence, whose services the Governors had used, died in April 1947. In June 1948 Robert Duncan Scott was appointed architect to the Governors, with an annual retaining fee of £5 [20]. Scott was soon busy with the eradication of the death watch beetle, which was found in the boardroom and the spiral staircase down from it, the common hall and guest chamber, and in some of the roof timbers. The cost was £577. Repairs involving the use of scaffolding were carried out in 1951, repointing and the painting of ironwork. Scott also gave thought to the development of hospital property, so that it would bring in a larger income. When Clark's College left the Old Cloth Hall, he considered that it might become a factory. He suggested that the garden front in North Street could be used for shops with offices over them. No use other than that could be found for 22 High Street, where the lease expired in 1950. It was not renewed until June 1953, for seven years from Christmas 1952, for £650 a year.

Abbot's Hospital Guildford

The chaplain, A.L. Gardiner, died in March 1950. He was succeeded by S.H. Courtnay Smith, a former curate of Holy Trinity who had retired from the rectory of Elstead. His payment was fixed at £30. Once again the Charity Commissioners objected to a sum of more than £10. They were persuaded to allow £30 for Smith, but insisted that it must not be given to his successor. Smith died in July 1952. The Reverend C.C. Pearson, an elderly curate at Holy Trinity, most of whose ministry had been in Bengal, offered to undertake the chaplaincy without pay. This was accepted, but Pearson resigned early in 1953. The Governors debated whether a chaplain was necessary, as there were five clergymen at Holy Trinity and St Mary. Nonetheless, the Reverend H.C. Hargeaves was appointed. In 1952, when the benefice of Holy Trinity was vacant, the sequestrators asked for the statutory payment by the hospital of thirty shillings to be restored, and this was agreed. R.S.B Sinclair, who had succeeded Southam as Rector and Provost in 1937, had not accepted it.

In 1951 discussion is recorded about the need of changes in the management of the hospital, especially the possibility of appointing a married master in the future. The Charity Commissioners recommended delay, as changes would require an Act of Parliament, but the Governors decided to ask for a new scheme, and appointed a subcommittee to prepare a draft. Archbishop Fisher's approval had been secured. The Act of Parliament was dated 14 July 1953. Most of the alterations were to make the transaction of business more straightforward, and to suit changed circumstances. The most significant changes were these.

1. The senior aldermen and councillors on the governing body were replaced by four representative Governors, all to be members of the Church of England, appointed by the Borough Council, but not necessarily members of the Council. There were to be five co-optative Governors, with no residential qualifications. The first four of these were named in the Act, Lawrence Powell, Arthur John Bradford Green, Arthur Williams and William George Lamport Sheppard, all of them non-official Governors under the 1861 scheme.
2. The Governors were given more freedom to make decisions.
3. The area of benefit was defined as "the Borough of Guildford as constituted from time to time".
4. No minimum age was stated for the master or residents, who were to number twenty-two, and there was no stated proportion of men to women.
5. No mention was made of the master's matrimonial state - or specifically of his being male.
6. The annual payment of £1.10s to the Rector of Holy Trinity was abolished, and was compounded by the transfer of £60 $2^1/_2$% consols to the Church Commissioners as part of the endowment capital of the benefice.

The Reformed Community

7. No payment to the residents was mentioned.

8. No provision was made for a chaplain, but the appointment could be covered by "such other officers as the Governors consider expedient for the superintendence and care of the Alms-persons".

9. Not less than £200 was to be paid yearly to the Official Trustee of Charitable Funds, to be invested for the extraordinary repair fund.

The first meeting after the Act of Parliament was on 7 October 1953, for which a new minute book was opened. The Mayor, Donald Wilkins, was elected chairman, by existing custom, and the appointments of the clerk, nurse, porter and assistant nurse were confirmed

The coronation of Queen Elizabeth II was celebrated on 2 June 1953. The Governors accepted the offer by R. Porter & Co. Ltd to lend and install a television set for the occasion. It was fixed up in the common hall, and was much appreciated. The idea was put forward to restore the lawns in the lower garden to commemorate the coronation, but it was defeated, even though the potatoes grown there were not of good quality. Then there was a change of mind, and the vegetable gardens gave place to grass before the coronation. [21]

The consideration, in 1951, of the advantages of having a married master was not entirely theoretical. Wale had been in office for twenty-four years, and reached his eighty-second birthday in September. Archbishop Fisher approved of the appointment of a married man, and so the qualification of being single was not included in the 1953 scheme, as has been noted above. As the master's strength and ability waned, the clerk, R.H. Percy, took more responsibility for day-to-day decisions, and this led to his having the hospital virtually under his very efficient but firm control. Percy discussed the situation with the Charity Commission. There was no statutory provision made for removing a master, other than for misconduct, even if he became incompetent through age or infirmity. If Wale stayed until he died, should an assistant be appointed to do the work; or could authority be given for his retirement with a pension? In May 1951 the Commission replied that a pension of £4 a week would be approved, but suggested that Wale should become a brother, and remain where he was known. By the end of 1953 the master was no longer able exert authority, and there were suspicions that some of the brothers were drinking, and playing cards. Wale was worried about his future. His only private income was a small pension from the Guild of Servants of the Sanctuary. He did not want to move into a brother's room, as he would be sensitive to the loss of standing, but he would be prepared to go into the room prepared for the assistant nurse, but not used. By February 1954 Percy had succeeded in assuring him that he could retire safely, with a pension of £3, with free fuel and the room that he asked for. Ernest Wale retired in May. The Governors decided to give a book, and he chose, characteristically, the abridged edition of the *Anglican Missal*. Later in the year the residents and staff subscribed to present him with a table reading stand. He lived on in the hospital until the beginning of

Abbot's Hospital Guildford

1958, and died in Mount Alvernia Hospital on 18 January. His burial was preceded by a requiem at St Nicolas'.

1. For St Cross Hospital Winchester and the Earl of Guilford see Martin 1962.
2. See Smith 1939, pp 881-887 for the hospital and manufacture.
3. The 1861 scheme is printed as appendix 4.
4. The normal term for the corporate body was always "The Master and Brethren". It is doubtful whether the sisters ever had any formal part in the business of the hospital.
5. The government of Guildford by the Mayor and the Approved Men was ended by the Municipal Corporations Act 1835. The new corporation first met on I January 1836.
6. See chapter 3, p 38.
7. I owe this anecdote to Mr F.H.G. Percy, archivist of Whitgift School. There is no complete list of wardens of Whitgift's Hospital.
8. Mangles had been Liberal Member of Parliament for Guildford 1841-1858. His name is consistently misspelt 'Donelly' in the hospital minutes.
9. Birch's bequest was subsequently regarded as part of the endowment of the hospital, and has been separately mentioned in schemes of management.
10. William Hillier Onslow, first Earl.
11. The master's journal for 1 April 1891 records "Revd H.C.Gaye. Kindly administered the Sacrement to two Sisters, and five Brothers", presumably not in the chapel.
12. The accompanying patten was made by Walter Keith in 1894, to match the chalice. In 1925 the base of the chalice was enlarged by Barkentin and Krall, to make it more stable. The cost was £5.
13. The money was repaid in thirteen years.
14. The five volumes of Palmer's summaries and analyses of the hospital records are now kept at Lambeth Palace Library (MSS 1410-14).
15. Thomas Riley Clemence later designed the municipal offices in the upper High Street, now demolished.
16. The budget for 1909 allowed £1,200,000 for the pensions which could be received by those over 70, whose other income did not exceed ten shillings. The pension was five shillings, but married couples had to share 7/6d.
17. At this meeting it was decided that the archives of the hospital should be catalogued by Miss D.L. Powell of the Surrey Record Office, for a charge of £15. They were taken by motor car to the Public Record Office on 23 July 1927. The list was published in *Records of Schools and Other Endowed Institutions* issued by the Surrey County Council in 1930, pp 50-84.

The Reformed Community

18. In the hospital records at this time the stable was often referred to as the Cloth Hall. To avoid confusion that name is not used for it in this book.

19. In July 1940 the Governors resolved that the railings might be given to the government "for munition work". In 1942 this was repeated, if the Rector and church wardens agreed. They were taken away in 1943.

20. Duncan Scott, in the later partnership Scott Brownrigg & Turner, was responsible for many prominent buildings in Guildford in the 1960s, among them the Yvonne Arnaud Theatre. They also designed Hillier House, the flats in Farnham Road replacing the Onslow Almshouses.

21. Those who objected in the 1970s to the alleged destruction of Archbishop Abbot's Jacobean garden must have been ignorant of its recent history.

Abbot's Hospital Guildford

SIX
MODERN TIMES

When the vacancy at Trinity Hospital was advertised there were eighty-four applications. Six were chosen for interview, and on 14 April 1954 the Governors' unanimous choice was Major John Mostyn, a married man, whose working life had been in the education service. After one year as an assistant master in Sussex he became a headmaster in Wales, but after one year, in 1914, he left for the army, and was commissioned in the Royal Welch Fusiliers. After the war he lectured at Saltley College Birmingham, and then, from 1926 to 1952, was Director of Education for Radnorshire. Mostyn became master of the hospital on 1 June. He had a motor car, and was given permission to keep it by the porter's cottage, so long as it did not keep the light from the windows. A few months later a shelter was built for the vehicle.

When Donald Wilkins reached the end of his two years as Mayor in 1954, his successor, Leslie Codd, was not elected as chairman of the Governors. Instead Albert Puttock, Mayor from 1949 to 1952 was chosen. Puttock was chairman until 1963, when he was succeeded by Geoffrey Osborn Swayne. It was decided that the new master should attend the second part of Governors' meetings, when business that was not his concern had been concluded.

In April 1954 the Governors made a decision that brought about a radical change in the financial position of the residents. The weekly payment, by then twelve shillings, was no longer required by the new scheme, and it was abolished. Instead a gift of twenty-six shillings would be made at Christmas. Those who qualified were encouraged to apply for National Assistance.

Clark's College left the Old Cloth Hall at the end of 1954, and re-opened the school in the Portsmouth Road. Messrs Cow & Gate Ltd applied for the use of the building, and were granted a lease from 25 September for twenty-one years, for the annual charge of £600.

In 1955 some minor repairs were done by the tenant of 22 High Street, during which it was found that the front of the building was badly decayed. Responsibility for major repairs lay with the Governors, who made the structure safe, but began to consider re-building the property. In 1958 Grove asked for a new, long lease, with the intention of erecting some lock-up shops in Jeffries Passage, and later rebuilding the front of the shop. In the meanwhile Percy had discovered, as Grove seems to have assumed, that the whole of the wall of 22 High Street on its west side belonged to number 22, and that the Governors had the right to put doors and windows in it. A small store by the end of the number 22 land was bought in 1958 for £150 to increase the hospital holding. Later, in 1959, A. Grove (Guildford) Ltd received compensation for the balance of the term of the lease, after leaving the premises. The decision had been made to build a new shop to the designs of Duncan Scott. The demolition was carried out by Ebenezer Mears Contractors Ltd, for £570, and the contract for the new building was given to R. Holford, whose estimate was £18,822. The price rose to £21,500, which was found by selling stock, the value to be replaced over twenty-one years. A twenty-one year lease to Messrs Importers Tea Stores Limited was granted from 25 March 1961. In May the tenant sublet the rear of the premises as a lock-up shop in Jeffries Passage to R.F.H. Porter, trading as A. Grove & Co Ltd. By February 1964 this business had come to an end, and Porter was given permission to sublet to Crown Appliances Limited.

An extra room for a sister was made in 1954 by dividing the kitchen, as an ordinary room was needed for an assistant nurse. This cost £125. A further £632.6s was spent in 1955 on a new range in the kitchen, improvements to the bathroom and lavatory accommodation, some modernising of the master's kitchen, and the installing of an upstairs lavatory in his quarters. All this money came from the extraordinary repair fund, as did £85.12s for repairing leaded lights. In 1956 the bell turret was repaired, and the clock was examined by Geoffrey Stevens, who was appointed to care for it, and did so for many years.

Mostyn carried out his duties understandingly, discovering the ways in which the routine was enlivened in the small community. In 1955 one sister was fetching coal with the light of a candle, when her scarf caught fire. The master reported that no damage had been done to the sister or the coal but that the scarf had been completely charred. He suggested that candles should be banned, and electric torches supplied, at a cost of £3.5s. In 1957 he received a gift of knitted shoulder wraps for the sisters, which were much appreciated. By this time the clerk, R.H. Percy, had taken responsibility for annual gaudy nights, which developed into refreshments followed by entertainments, to which residents from other almshouses were invited. Mostyn also knew very well that the hospital provided accommodation and facilities that were below the standard that should be considered desirable. In November 1957 he made some moderate suggestions, which were agreed to - better lighting in the main entrance, on the staircases and by the sinks, and the placing of sinks on the ground floor, so that dirty water need not be carried upstairs to be poured away. His request for a bath in the cellar for the sisters was not approved. Washbasins were put into sisters' rooms on the ground floor in 1958, and given to the men in 1959.

The decision was made in 1960 by the Charity Commission that married people separated from their spouses could not be regarded as single, and so were not eligible for admission to the hospital.

The consecration of the Cathedral on 17 May 1961 caused Holy Trinity to revert to parochial status alone. The last Provost, Walter Boulton, resigned, and was succeeded as Rector in 1962 by Michael Warwick Hocking. H.C. Hargreaves, the chaplain, had resigned in 1961. At his first attendance at a Governors' meeting, on 25 April 1962,

Modern Times

Hocking said that he expected that he would be the chaplain, and since then the appointment has been held by him and by his successors in the rectory. A service was held in Holy Trinity on 29 October 1962 to mark the four hundredth anniversary of George Abbot's birth. Archbishop Ramsey and his predecessor G.F. Fisher were in turn invited to preach, but could not come. As no other notable person could be found, the sermon was preached by Hocking, who had already begun to shew a keen interest in the hospital's affairs.

Early in 1962 alterations to the lavatories and the cellar stairs were considered, but nothing was done, nor were repairs to the master's quarters carried out. External work was considered more important, and repairs were done to roofs, walls and windows, and to the main entrance and the front balustrade, the estimates, including scaffolding, being £3447.14s. In 1942 it had been reported that the wooden front gates were rotting away. They remained until 1962, when they were replaced with iron gates designed by Duncan Scott, costing £200. They were hung in February 1964. Scott also designed new railings for the northern end of the hospital garden. These cost £946, and began to be put up in April 1963, replacing those taken away during the war.[1] This ironwork was made by Sex & Son of Send. All this work was paid for from the extraordinary repair fund, which stood at £4500.

At the turn of the year, 1962-3, Hocking and Mostyn discussed the state of the hospital's facilities, and the lack of many applications from men for admission. The conversation became known to the Governors, and caused a stir at their January meeting, at which Hocking defended the criticisms that he had made. At the February meeting a subcommittee was formed, and reported in March. A ten-year plan was recommended, with these aims: all rooms should have washbasins and draining-boards immediately; small refrigerators should be provided; baths and showers should be considered; central heating should be hoped for; the floors of upstairs rooms should be raised, so that the residents could look out of the windows when sitting down. The subcommittee had also considered other suggestions: the provision of breakfast, communal meals, and alterations so that married couples could be admitted to two-room flats, but all these were considered impossible. It was noted that the residents said that they were happy to cook on their stoves and be warmed by them. The Governors decided to obtain estimates for all the work that the subcommittee had recommended, with central heating as the main priority. Instead, sinks were fitted, with splash-boards, all of which cost £532. Twenty-one refrigerators were bought in October, for £296.

At the Governors' meeting in November 1963, Percy presented a statement estimating the cost of the work that the Governors wished to undertake at not much less than £10,000. He then opened the question of charging the residents rent, suggesting twenty-five shillings a week. The following week there was another meeting, on 27 November, attended by the General Secretary of the National Association of Almshouses. He explained that supplementary payments could be claimed by right, so that residents should be persuaded not to have "poor law" qualms. He advised that although the National Assistance Board would consider that payments by residents to the hospital would be rent, the Governors should not use that word, to avoid the risk of establishing a landlord/tenant relationship. Instead the payments should be called contributions. He agreed that £1.5s would be a suitable figure, and said that the income would make improvements to the hospital possible. The Governors decided unanimously to charge contributions and the first were received on 2 March 1964. Those brothers and sisters who needed assistance were helped to apply for supplementary payments. Since the principle of payment for accommodation in the hospital, subsidised when necessary from public funds, was accepted, the practice has continued, and has provided a significant proportion of the hospital's income.

The improvements continued, under the supervision of Duncan Scott. The refrigerators were installed in December 1963, and this led to the discovery that the electrical wiring was overloaded, and must be corrected. The purchase of small electric cookers and fires, (with simulated glowing coal) and the wiring and plug points, with the rewiring for the refrigerators, and the provision of slot meters, cost £3342.18.1d. The installation of central heating began in June 1964, and included the boardroom and the master's quarters. The cost was £5541.8.1d. To assist in the payment for the improvements, the Governors realised £3500 of the endowment capital, to be replaced over fifteen years. Scott remained consulting architect until his death in 1971.

In 1964, one of the brothers, G.B. Gloyne, gave a Jacobean chest, for the chapel. Later in the same year a large sixteenth century German chest was given by John Burt. In January 1965 a bequest of £500 from Captain Holroyd was announced. It was later increased to £1203.19.5d. The Governors gave £50 to the former nurse, Miss Oates, and set up a subcommittee to make suggestions for the balance. It was decided to improve important parts of the hospital, as well as having a number of the pictures cleaned. The guest hall was given carpets, new lighting and twelve chairs. The boardroom was also recarpeted, and an eighteenth century brass six-branch chandelier was bought, and wired for electric candles. The common hall was also relit.

Gowns and hats were still worn at this time, and in 1967 six sets were bought for £93.13s.

The master reported in 1965 that there had been much talk in the hospital about television. He took a vote in the chapel, and twelve out of the fourteen present said that they would like one in the common hall. The Governors agreed to pay for the rental. By 1969 it was no longer needed, as all who wanted to watch it had sets in their own rooms.

R.H. Percy announced in 1965 that he was shortly to leave the solicitors' firm Smallpeice & Merriman, and would become full-time clerk to the magistrates. Up till then secretarial and accounting work had been done in the firm's office; now he would need assistance for about eight hours a week, at ten shillings an hour. This was agreed.

In June 1965, Cow & Gate indicated that they wished to assign the balance, ten years, of their lease of the Old Cloth Hall. The County Council, with the Borough Council, were interested in using the building. However, Cow & Gate assigned the lease to the Star and Garter Homes. Subsequently Star and Garter sublet the building to the Surrey County Council, to house the Justices' offices and the probation office.

Mostyn was a popular master. In 1967 he and his wife celebrated their golden wedding. To mark this, Gloyne raised a collection from the residents to pay for the painting of the master's portrait by Graham Mervyn, and it was presented to him and Mrs Mostyn at a ceremony in the common hall.

The three hundredth anniversary of the hospital was kept in 1969, with a service in Holy Trinity, when Hocking preached. Afterwards there was a reception in the hospital grounds. Residents from Hillier House and the Lovejoy and Stoke charities attended as guests.

In February 1971 Mostyn, who was approaching eighty, announced that he wished to retire. The Governors had already been thinking about accommodation for him, and it was decided to have two rooms in the south-west corner adapted to provide a sitting room, bedroom, kitchen and bathroom. He was given a pension and the flat rent-free. Mostyn's retirement took effect on 31 May 1972. He retained the flat for the rest of his life, happily describing himself as the pastmaster. He died in south Wales on 23 May 1983.

A subcommittee was formed to look for a new master. The appointment was advertised in *The Times* and the *Surrey Advertiser*, and there were ninety-five applicants, five of whom were interviewed on 17 March. The subcommittee's choice was recommended to the Governors, who, on 30 March appointed John Wallace Stockwood Fogwill, a married man, who had lived in Guildford since 1939. He was director and secretary of Fogwills Ltd, corn, coal and seed factors, a long-established family business, until it closed in 1966. He then worked for a London estate agent, managing the property of the Haberdashers' Company and other charities. He arrived to take the appointment at 9.30 a.m. on 1 June 1972.

The Governors' meeting on 26 September 1974 included a discussion of a report by the clerk. Percy pointed out that he had been associated with the hospital longer than any of the Governors or residents. He therefore was well aware of the significance of the fact that a sister's room had been vacant for some time - the first time that this had ever happened. He attributed the lack of applicants to the poor standard of accommodation provided in the hospital. The Governors did not shew much alarm at that stage. Possibly they hoped that the Local Government Act, which had come into effect on 1 April, would increase the number of applicants from the much enlarged borough of Guildford. This hope was not borne out, and the difficulty in filling the hospital was one of the reasons for the development plans that were to be formed.

In the evening of 5 October 1974 the hospital was shaken by the bomb that exploded in the Horse and Groom public house in North Street. The master, with the porter and nurse, went to see if any help was needed, but there was nothing for them to do. The following day detectives visited the hospital, and took statements from all the residents.

The silver jubilee of Queen Elizabeth II in 1977 was marked by visits of members of the royal family to towns throughout the country. Princess Anne came to Guildford on 6 July and spent twenty minutes in the hospital.

When the Star and Garter lease of the Old Cloth Hall expired at Christmas 1975, the Surrey County Council took a new lease for fifteen months. The new law courts were complete by December 1976, and the Justices' clerk's office moved there, leaving the Old Cloth Hall empty, as the County Council had no further use for the building. The Governors sought a new tenant, or some other use for the premises, which were extensively repaired, partly at the Council's expense. Some community use was thought possible, and some considered that a town centre comprehensive school might need the space. The *Surrey Advertiser* was approached, but the staff considered that it was too far from their premises in Martyr Road. Finally Laura Ashley Ltd were given a lease for twenty-five years from 25 March 1978, and began trading on 7 September 1979.

In 1973 the architect David Nye was asked to make a survey of the hospital, and to make suggestions for the best use of the buildings. His early notions included redesigning the interior of the Old Cloth Hall to make sixteen offices, that would produce an annual income of £11,000 from an outlay of about £40,000. This suggestion was not followed up, as has been shewn. He also suggested building flats and shops along Jeffries Passage, on the land occupied by the cottage and carpark. This idea was also not pursued. Regarding the hospital building he said that financial stress had led to a policy of dealing with defects as they arose. This would be possible for another ten to fifteen years, but it would be more economical to have a proper plan of maintenance and repair. He reported that there was death watch beetle and furniture beetle in structural timbers, that much brickwork needed repointing, and that major repairs were needed in the leadwork of the turrets and the guttering. The lead on the turrets was repaired in 1977.

David Nye was also asked to consider the construction of extra accommodation in the garden. He spoke of a three storey building at the North Street end, to secure the privacy of the garden. This could give either twenty-two single flats, with shared bathrooms, or ten flats for two people, each with its bathroom and lavatory. Discussion of various proposals continued into 1976, and had to take the lack of applicants for the hospital rooms into consideration. Percy suggested that two-room flats could be made in the courtyard wings. This would be more attractive, though it would halve the accommodation. In June the Governors were moving towards trying to build sufficient rooms in the garden for all the brothers and sisters, but then wondered what the old rooms could be used for. Suggestions included barristers' chambers, sixth form rooms for the Royal Grammar School, or some use by the University of Surrey or the College of Law. It was realised that planning permission for a building in the garden might be refused, and thought was given to an alternative site. Nonetheless, Nye was asked to prepare elevations for a garden building, so that an application could be made for outline planning permission.

In February 1977 the present writer suggested that a solution to the problem of the courtyard could be found by turning each staircase of four rooms into a house. This was adopted, and David Nye prepared plans. It was decided that these houses should not be for letting to produce income, but allocated to married couples. For this the scheme of management would need to be altered.

The prolonged discussion of the hospital's development could not be kept secret. There was curiosity, and among some there was instinctive hostility. At the request of the Guildford Society a public meeting was held on 7 November 1977, when Nye and Percy explained the proposals. By this time much opposition had been declared, and ventilated in the *Surrey Advertiser* by individuals and by those who spoke on behalf of the Guildford Society and the Holy Trinity Amenity Group. It was noted that most of the criticisms were concerned solely with the appearance of the exterior of the old building, which the Governors did not intend to alter in any way, and with the need to preserve the garden, which was scarcely ever visited or looked at. Very little thought was expressed for the comfort and needs of the residents - or for the growing number of empty rooms - three by the end of 1977. R.H. Percy devoted much time to careful public explanation of what the Governors hoped to achieve, answering the criticisms, both reasonable and unreasonable. Councillor John Boyce, one of the Governors, also played a very significant part in the story, as he was able to provide a trusted link between the Governors and the Borough Council and its officials.

John Fogwill's service as master was not long. During 1977 his health deteriorated, and his resignation became necessary. The brothers and sisters appreciated his personal care for them, which made it possible for some of them to remain in their rooms when sickness or infirmity could have taken them to hospital. He left on 26 July 1978 and retired on 31 July. He died in his own home in Guildford on 6 April 1979.

The vacancy of the mastership was advertised in *The Times* and the *Surrey Advertiser*, and two applicants were interviewed. The Governors' choice was for Gerard Taylor, who had served in the Royal Marines, and then been bursar of the Perse School Cambridge and of Frensham Heights School. Archbishop Coggan's approval was given, and he took up the appointment on 1 August 1978. With his wife he moved into a community that was uncertain about the future, and overshadowed by controversy. During his service he cared for the residents through revolutionary changes, and with the additional distraction of large-scale builders' work, continued year after year.

Before the end of 1977 the Borough Council had been persuaded that a building in the hospital garden was the only solution to the problem of providing accommodation for the residents of a standard suitable for modern times. There was not yet agreement about the exact position or size of the proposed building. Because of the large amount of public interest, and the level of opposition, the Secretary of State for the Environment,

Abbot's Hospital Guildford

Peter Shore, intervened. With powers derived from the Town and Country Planning Act 1971 he ordered the Borough Council to take no action until he had decided whether or not to reserve the decision regarding planning permission to himself. He did make that decision and it was announced that there would be a public enquiry.

The Secretary of State appointed W.A. Greenoff to be the inspector for the enquiry, which opened in Guildford on 4 April 1979, and lasted two days. The Governors were represented by Michael Fitzgerald of Counsel, with John Leslie of Triggs Turner as their solicitor.[2] The Borough Council was represented, to support the Governors' application. Evidence was given on behalf of the Governors by their clerk, the master, David Nye the architect, and by J.M. Scott, the General Secretary of the National Association of Almshouses. Objections were heard from those bodies which had declared their opposition, and from some individuals. The inspector's site inspection was delayed by his illness, but took place on 14 May. Furthermore, some anxiety was caused by the change of government following the general election, held shortly after the public enquiry. When Mr Greenoff's report was issued, it was seen that he had recommended that planning permission and listed building consent should be granted to the Governors. He said that the hospital, by reason of its location, size and shape, made a valuable contribution to the High Street and North Street, and that although it was within a conservation area, it was well placed for old people at the centre of a busy, thriving old-established town, where much of the character derived from intensive use and tightly packed buildings. The new Secretary of State, Michael Heseltine, granted the necessary permission and consents on 3 December 1979.

Preparations for the new building took a long time. David Nye retired from his practice in August 1981. The Governors appointed Nye, Saunders & Partners to be their architects, and the senior partner, Arthur Saunders, agreed to use the plans prepared by Nye.

On 8 August 1981, Miss Jane Farley, one of the sisters, celebrated her hundredth birthday, and seventy people attended her party. She was the first known member of the hospital community to become a centenarian.[3]

In 1982 new leases were prepared for 165 (formerly 22) High Street, and for 16 Jeffries Passage for twenty years from 25 March. These were with Importers Retail Salerooms Ltd and Crown Electrical (Guildford) respectively.

On 6 April 1983 a gaudy was held, the first for several years, and took the form of a dinner in the common hall for the residents and the Governors. On the following Monday, 11 April, work began on the new building. The contractors who had been appointed were E.C. Hughes Ltd, but they had been absorbed by Wiltshier Ltd (Reading). A commemoration stone was laid by the Lord Lieutenant of Surrey, Lord Hamilton of Dalzell, at a small ceremony on 12 August 1983. In his speech Lord Hamilton said that he regretted the rise in the cost of the total work caused by the objections that had been raised, in "the splendidly democratic machinery which proposals of this sort set in motion".

Modern Times

Work went on through the winter, and there was a topping out on 14 March 1984, when the master laid the final tile on the roof. Some of the brothers and sisters moved into their new homes on 6 September, even though there were some omissions and shortcomings -clear glass in the bathroom windows, for example. There are twelve flats, each with living room and bedroom, kitchen, bathroom and lavatory. A lift was installed, to carry people from the lower, garden level to the old courtyard. The cost of the building, and the lift, including fees, was £430,173. The Governors were assisted by the Housing Corporation with a grant of £264,842, and a loan of £73,693, repayable over sixty years

Before the flats were occupied, Geoffrey Swayne, who had been a Governor for thirty-five years, died on 16 April. In his place the Governors elected John Fergrieve Brown as chairman. He had been a Governor since 1957.

In 1985 two changes were made in the scheme of management. The parish of Stoke had been held in plurality with St Saviour's Guildford since 1974. In 1976 a united benefice was formed, St Saviour with Stoke-next-Guildford, and its Rector was named as a Governor, The other change was to remove the requirement that brothers and sisters should be single. They were now defined as "poor persons of good character". These alterations came into effect on 20 December. The first married couple to benefit from life in the hospital, apart from married masters and porters and their wives, were Edward and Mavis Wink, who arrived on 18 August 1986.

Rex Percy gave notice that he would retire on 5 December 1985, after forty years as clerk. Earlier in 1985 the oak doors and their overthrow in the archway of the new building were given by Percy and his wife, to mark his long association with the hospital. A dinner was held in Rex Percy's honour on 5 December.[4] John Leslie was appointed to succeed him.

Three pear trees were planted in the hospital grounds on 8 January 1986, as a reminder of the founder's coat of arms. Repairs and redecorating in the chapel were carried out, assisted in part by a grant from the Borough Council. After two Archbishops of Canterbury who did not visit the hospital, A.M. Ramsey and F.D. Coggan, Archbishop Runcie came to Guildford on 23 May 1986. During his stay he came to the hospital and made unhurried visits to the residents in their rooms, and met the Governors.

The next stage in bringing the hospital up to an acceptable standard was the conversion of the single rooms in the front courtyard into more spacious homes - four houses and two flats, as well as the quarters for the retired master. This was carried out by L.T. Deeprose Ltd, under the direction of the architect Arthur Saunders. Work began on 15 August 1988, and occupation was taken up in July 1989. The 1939 doors to the staircases were made like those they replaced, in two leaves, to open in the middle. They were now joined together, to hang as single doors. The cost of what was called the rehabilitation was £331,110, including fees. The Housing Corporation made a grant of £116,267, and a loan was raised from the Nationwide Building Society.

Abbot's Hospital Guildford

In 1989 the benefice of St Saviour's with Stoke-next-Guildford was divided into the two parishes from which it had been formed in 1976. At the request of the incumbents the governorship was attached to St John's Stoke, and the Rector, Stephen Sizer, joined the board. The amendment to the scheme was dated 29 May 1991.

Laura Ashley Ltd moved to other premises in North Street on 24 August 1990. While the Old Cloth Hall was unoccupied, in February 1991, there was a serious water leak, which caused much damage to the building. The lease was assigned on 4 July 1991 to The Edinburgh Woollen Mill Ltd, who opened for business shortly afterwards.

From April 1991 to January 1992 builders were again in the hospital. The Lexiconi Restoration & Development Company Limited carried out extensive repairs to the old roofs and chimneys. The cost was £179,832, including fees and value added tax. The Guildford Borough Council made a grant of £50,000, and £40,000 was received from English Heritage. From March to July 1992 repairs were done to the clock by F.F. Hill of Godalming, including the remaking of the striking hammer.

Gerard Taylor retired on 31 July 1992, and moved with his wife into the rooms in the south-west corner. His fourteen years in office saw more changes in the hospital than any other period since it was founded, changes both in the building and the additions to it, and in the community, with the introduction of married couples.[5] He also assumed more responsibility for day-to-day affairs than his immediate predecessors had been given. On this occasion the position was not advertised, and the Governors appointed John Moss, a retired schoolmaster who had taught in England, Tanzania and New Zealand. Improvements were made to the lodgings by the Lexconi Company, costing £29,055, and the new master, whose appointment had been approved by the Governors on 27 February, took up office on 1 August.

In 1992 the cost of running the hospital, discounting the repair work and interest on loans, was £74,286.

employees (salaries, wages, honoraria, national insurance)	31,638
estate costs (rates, insurance, garden, fuel, cleaning, routine repairs, architect's fees)	32,553
office expenses (postage, stationery, travel, telephone, audit etc.)	3,533
residents' expenses	607
transfer to extraordinary repair fund	1,785
transfer to cyclical maintenance fund	4,170
	£74,286

The ordinary income of the hospital that year was £117,870.

rents	63,500
investment income (less expenses, fees etc.)	11,053
West Wantley Farm annuity	12
residents' contributions	43,305
	£117,870

Modern Times

The final part of the programme begun in 1983 was undertaken in 1993, carried out by R.P. Harknett, New Stone & Restoration Co. Limited and Lexiconi. The cost amounted to £18,154, towards which grants were received from the Guildford Borough Council of £3,000, and from the Surrey Historic Buildings Trust Ltd of £1,000. The High Street front, which had looked shabby, was pointed where necessary, and other repairs were done to the structure, and to the doors and balustrade. Inside, the entrance area was decorated. Further back the divided staircase was made good, with new stone treads for the steps, the visible link between the upper and lower levels of the hospital, the old and the new.

1. In December 1954 an order was given for a wooden fence, to be supplied by Astolat for £17.4.4d.
2. I am grateful to Mr Lesie who has provided me with a summary account of the public enquiry.
3. Miss Farley died on 18 November 1982, aged 101.
4. Mr Percy died on 12 October 1991.
5. Mr Taylor was given the title of Master Emeritus by the Governors in May 1993. He died on 13 December 1997.

Abbot's Hospital Guildford

Appendix 1

MASTERS OF THE HOSPITAL

1. RICHARD ABBOTT — appointed 29 October 1622, died 2 March 1630

2. JASPER YARDLEY — appointed 24 March 1630, installed 25 March 1630, died 31 May 1639

3. HENRY SNELLING — elected and installed 31 May 1639, died 18 November 1643

4. THOMAS SMITH — elected and installed 18 November 1643, died 2 August 1644

5. HENRY HORNER — elected and installed 3 August 1644, died 9 February 1655

6. The Reverend JOHN HOLLAND MA — elected and installed 9 February 1655, died 6 July 1691

7. SAMUEL SHAW — elected and installed 6 July 1691, died 9 August 1702

8. SAMUEL BARTON — elected and installed 9 August 1702, died 12 October 1709

9. ROBERT BERRY — elected and installed 13 October 1709, died c 17 December 1719

10. THOMAS SANDS — elected and installed c 17 December 1719, died 17 June 1729

11. EPHRAIM WOOD — elected and installed 17 June 1729, died 2 May 1734

12. HENRY STOUGHTON — elected and installed 3 May 1734, died 27 July 1744

13. HUGH MOTH — elected and installed 27 July 1744, died 18 June 1749

14. WILLIAM GOODYER — elected and installed 18 June 1749, died 3 October 1762

Abbot's Hospital Guildford

15. The Reverend
    CORNELIUS JEALE BA
    elected 3 October 1762,
    commenced 4 October 1762,
    died 29 October 1762

16. MICHAEL WALLIS
    elected and installed 29 October 1762,
    died 12 March 1769

17. GEORGE LOVEDALE WHITE
    elected and installed 12 March 1769,
    died 18 May 1778

18. The Reverend
    EDMUND BREWER MA
    elected and installed 18 May 1778,
    died 22 February 1784

19. EDWARD BRINKWELL
    elected and Installed 23 February 1784,
    died 30 January 1792

20. RICHARD ELKINS
    elected and installed 30 January 1792,
    resigned 31 January 1809,
    died 29 March 1809

21. SAMUEL RUSSELL
    elected and installed 31 January 1809,
    died 8 May 1824

22. SAMUEL ROBINSON
    elected and installed 8 May 1824,
    died 1 May 1833

23. JESSE BOXALL
    elected and installed 1 May 1824,
    died 18 February 1846

24. ANDREW HOOKE
    elected and installed 18 February 1846,
    died 18 October 1853

25. GEORGE RUSSELL
    elected and installed 19 october 1853,
    died 9 August 1861

26. THOMAS TERRY
    appointed 12 October 1861,
    installed 28 October 1861,
    died 21 February 1885

27. GEORGE CHALLEN
    appointed 17 April 1885,
    commenced 27 April 1885,
    died 10 April 1890

28. HENRY HARRIS
    appointed 23 May 1890,
    commenced 19 June 1890,
    died 20 September 1913

Appendix 1

29. PHILIP GRIGGS PALMER appointed 4 November 1913,
  commenced 11 November 1913,
  died 13 December 1926

30. ERNEST GEORGE appointed 9 April 1927,
  REIGNOLDS WALE introduced 10 April 1927,
  resigned May 1954,
  died 18 January 1958

31. Major JOHN MOSTYN MC TD, MA appointed 21 April 1954,
  commenced 1 June 1954,
  resigned 31 May 1972,
  died 23 May 1983

32. JOHN WALLACE appointed 30 March 1972,
  STOCKWOOD FOGWILL commenced 1 June 1972,
  resigned 31 July 1978,
  died 6 April 1979

33. HENRY GERARD TAYLOR BEM appointed 27 April 1978,
  commenced 1 August 1978,
  resigned 31 July 1992
  died 13 December 1997

34. JOHN WALKER MOSS BSc appointed 27 February 1992,
  commenced 1 August.1992

Abbot's Hospital Guildford

Appendix 2

THE FIRST STATUTES

The Othe of the Kings Soueraigntie.

I. A.B. doe vtterly testifie & declare in my conscience, that the Kings highnesse is the onely supreme gouernor of this Realme, & of all other his Highnes Dominions & countries, as well in all spirituall or Ecclesiasticall things or causes, as temporall, & that no forraine Prince, person, prelate, State or Potentate, hath or ought to haue any iurisdiction, power, superioritie, preheminence or authoritie Ecclesiasticall or spirituall within this Realme, And therefore I doe vtterly renounce, & forsake all forren Jurisdictions, powes, superiorities and authorities: and doe promise that from henceforth, I shall beare faith & true allegiance to the Kings highnesse, his heires and lawful successors, and to my power shall assist & defend all Jurisdictions, priuiledges, preheminences and authorities, granted or belonging to the Kings highnes, his heires and successors, or vnited and annexed to the Imperiall Crowne of this Realme. so helpe me God, and the contents of this Booke.

THE FOVNDERS STATVTS
FOR THE GOOD GOVERNEMENT OF THE
Hospitall of the Blessed Trinitie, in Guildford.

THE PREFACE.

Forasmuch as euery Christian man is bounde, according to the measure of grace and mercy which he hath receaued from God, to render back againe to his Eternall Father, such tokens of gratefulnes and thankfulnes as are in his power; And I George Abbott Archbishop of Canterbury, from the meere mercy of that Blessed God (besides the inward graces of his holy Spiritt), hauing ben partaker of some earthly & worldly benefitts, more then most of my birth or ranke haue attayned vnto, I haue held it agreeable with my duetie, to leaue behind mee to posteritie, some monument of my thankefulnes to my Creator, and some testimony of my faith in Jesus Christ, which, if it bring not forth some fruite to his glory, is to be held but a dead and vnprofitable faith. And therefore my affection leading me to the Towne of Guildford, where I was borne, and where my aged Parents liued many years with good report, I haue thought vpon the erecting of an Hospitall there, which I haue dedicated to the Blessed Trinitie, and intending that poore people should be releeued therein, thinke good to lay downe certaine Statutes and Ordinances, which shall be for the gouverning of the Maister, Brethren and Sisters there, as also of all other persons who are therein to be placed; And for the guiding of the Possessions and Rents which God hath, and may enable me to bestow vppon the same. In the name therefore of the Father, the Sonne, and the holy Ghost, who direct my penne aright, I thus beginne.

Chap: 1:
Of the Maister of the Hospitall, and his Office or Duetie.

There can no Body be well governed, but there must be a Head to oversee and direct all the rest of the Members: This Head I appoint to be the *Maister*, whose office shall be to rule and governe all the rest, with mildenesse and love, if it may be, otherwise with moderate severitie, if there be just cause. He shall require and exact of the Brethren and Sisters the due observation of the Ordinances and Statutes: He shall keepe one key of the Common Chest, and another of the Evidence house, that nothing be there done without his privity. He shall cause the gates of the Hospitall to be opened and locked at due times appoynted, and night by night shall have the keyes brought vnto him. He shall be present when any one is admitted, and whensoever Wages or any allowances are to be payd. He shalbe carefull to preserve and defend the Landes and Inheritance of the Howse, and to that purpose shall see the Evidences well and safely layd up. He shall see that all

Entries be duely made in the Lidger Booke. He shall looke in tyme to Reparations, and all other good husbandry of the *Hospitall*, being carefull that no fire or candle be dangerously kept. If any lodging be voyd he shall keepe the key thereof till it be to be delivered to some Brother or Sister which is newly to be admitted.

Chap: 2:

Of the qualitie of the Maister.

This Maister of the Hospital I appoint to be a man fearing God, of good name and fame of Fifty yeares of age at the least; borne, or having lived Twentie yeares of age before in the Towne of Guildford, which I will have evermore to be vnderstood within that Compasse, which is governed by the Maior and no otherwise. He shall be at the tyme of his nomination or election, a single and vnmaried man, and so shall continew so long as he remayneth *Maister*. And if he thinke fitt to marry and doe so indeede, I appoint, that on perrill of breach of his oath he leave the place within three dayes, to a new Election or Nomination. If any person have ben Maior of the Towne and hath governed with good report he shalbe capable of this place, and so shall the Minister who is Parson of Trinitie Church in Guilford although he were not borne in the Towne, so that either of theis be single men, and furnished with the rest of the conditions named in this Chapter. He shalbe as neere as may be a pvident man, acquainted with affaires of the world, especially for letting and setting of Lande, or turning it to the best benefitt of the place where he is Maister.

Chap: 3:

Of the manner, how the Maister shall be chosen, or appointed.

I doe reserve vnto my selfe the Nominacion of this *Maister* so long as it pleaseth God that I shall live: And after my decease I appoint, that if the place shalbe voyd by the Death, Resignation, or Expulsion of the former Maister, that then the Vice-Maister, or, in his absence, the Senior Brother, shall as soon as may be, give notice to the Electors, that the place is voyd, that so they may meete together in the Chappell of the Hospitall to make a new Choice. The Electors I appoint to be Five. The Maior of Guildford, or in his absence, his Deputie. The Parson of Trinitie parish, or if he be not in towne, the Parson of St Nicholas Parish, and Three of the Brethren of the Hospitall; That is to say, the Vice-Maister, and the two Senior or most auncient Brethren: And looke on whom the greater part of theis Five shall agree, he shall be admitted to the place of the Maister. These shall proceede without favour or affection, or without any corruption whatsoever directly or indirectly as in the presence of God, who iudgeth righteously touching the good or evill actions of all men in the day of Christ. This Election I appoint to be within

Abbot's Hospital Guildford

fower and twentie howers of the being voyd of the Maistership, or at least within that space after that it shall be knowne that the place is voyd. And if within that time it be not supplyed by a new Election; I then order, that by way of Devolution it shall fall to the Archbishop of Canterbury, to be nominated by him according to my Statutes. And if the See of Canterbury be voyd or the Archbishop *sede plena*, shall not designe the Maister within twelve dayes, Then it shalbe in the Nomination of the Bishop of *Winton* for the time being; and if that See be also voyd, or the Bishop, *sede plena*, shall not appoint the Maister within seaven dayes, Then Sr George *More* of Loseley Knight, or after his decease, the Heire of his howse whosoever he shall be from time to time, shall have the sole appointing and Designeing of the Maister, which if it be not compleated within five dayes, the Choice shall returne to the first Electors. When the Election or Nomination is thus passed, the Person Elected or nominated shall in the presence of all the Brethren of the Howse, in the Chappell of the Hospitall, take first the Oath of Soveraigntie & Obedience unto the *Kings Maiestie*, his lawfull Heires and Successors as is by Law prescribed, and then this Oath here ensuing. *I. A.B. from henceforth, as long as I shall continue and remaine Maister of this Hospitall, shall and will by Gods assistance doe my best endeauour, to performe, fulfill and obey, the Statuts, Ordinances & Constitutions of the same, so farre forth as they concerne me; and shall doe my best, that the rest of the Brethren and Sisters, as also all other, that are vnder me, doe keepe and obserue the same. I shall not hereafter at any time, procure, or willingly giue assent vnto the hurt, indaungering, or indomaging of the sayd Hospitall in the Hereditaments, or any the mooueable goods thereof, or in any thing that may concerne the State or welfaire thereof: but to my best skill and power, shall defend, promote and sett forward, the benefitt and commodite thereof while I liue. So me God in Christ Jesus.*

Chap: 4:

Of the Vice-Maister.

The Maister, end the Five Senior Brethren that be at home, shall, the morrow after Michaelmas day yearely, choose a Vice-Maister, one of the gravest and of best understanding, who shall governe in the absence of the Maister as is prescribed in theis Statutes: and the rest of the Brethren and Sisters shall, for that yeare, yeeld a regard and due respect unto him. The Election shall be made by the Maior part, where the Maister's voyce shall be accounted for two. At the end of the yeare, he shall have, as a Stipend, Thirteene Shillings and Fowerpence, out of the common Chest. He shall keepe one of the keyes of the Evidence howse, and another key of the common Chest; And in the absence of the Maister, he shall night by night have the keyes of the *Hospitall* brought vnto him.

Appendix 2

Chap: 5:

*Of the poore Brethren & Sisters, who
are capeable of that place.*

The *Head*, being thus setled, the Members are to be added, which must compleate the Body. On the right side I put the poore men, whom I call Brethren, and on the left side the poore weomen, whom I terme Sisters. I Ordaine that such as are to be nominated into these places, be persons of good name and fame: Noe Drunkards, or noted for contention; no Leapers, or such as haue any Contagious, infectious, or incureable Disease; None such as at any time haue ben knowne to have begged from doore to doore; But such as in their younger yeares have honestly laboured; and by age, impotency, or other hand of God, be growne poore, or fallen to decay; Such onely as haue ben borne in the Towne of *Guilford*, or have lived there, at the least, for Twenty yeares before; I will that they be Threescore years of age before they be chosen, single and vnmaried persons, and so to remaine, els, if they do afterward marry, by vertue of their Oath, they are to leave the *Hospitall*, and all interest they haue therein, within twoe dayes. And among, these, I would have preferred, such as have borne office, or haue ben good Traders in the Towne, whereby they have set other on worke, if any of them be fallen into povertie; Such as have ben souldiers, sent or chosen out of Guilford, and haue adventured their lives, or lost their blood for their Prince and Countrey; And if any be of my kinred or have served my Father, or mee, I would haue them to be capeable, although they were not borne in Guilford, nor be of the age aboue named, so that at one time there be not aboue Three of my kinred, or more then Three at once that haue ben my Servants: And so that otherwise they be qualifyed as before.

Chap: 6:

*The manner of choosing the
Brothers & Sisters.*

The nomination of these, during my life, I reserve vnto myselfe, but after my decease I appoint that the first place which falleth voyd by it of Brother or Sister, be filled and named by the Maior of Guildford, or in his absence by his Deputie, and the second place by the Maister of the Hospitall, or in his absence by the Schoole-Maister of the Free-Schoole in Guildford, and so turne after turne, the Third by the Maior or his Deputy, the Fourth by the Maister, or Schoole-Maister and so forward for ever. I doe ordaine that this nomination be perfited and accomplished within Fower and Twenty howers after the knowne death or avoydance of any formerly possessed wth the place: And if the Maior or his Deputie, for their turnes, do not designe the person to be supplyed within the space aboue named; Then my will is, That the Parson of the parish of St Nicholas do appoint him or her that is to succeede; And if the Maister of the *Hospitall*, or the Schoole-maister, do not designe for their turnes the person to be supplyed by them within the space afore-named, Then my will is, that the Parson of Trinitie parish do appoint him or her that is to succeede, if the sayd Parson be not at that time the Maister of the *Hospitall*, which if he be, Then the Nomination shall fall to the Parson of St Mareys Church in Guildford. All which Nominations I would have to be as in the presence of God, without Corruption or filthie lucre, without favour or sinister affection. For I give unto these persons this power onely vpon trust, and not to make a gaine of that, which I have spared from my back, and from my belly, and from my kinred, or from some other good use in some other place, to bestow for Gods sake, on the poore Members of *Christ* in this Towne. The Lord forbid, that any man should abuse this my Charitie, for which he did never sweat or labour. The manner of these Nominations I ordaine to be; That the Maior, Maister of the *Hospitall*, or other person in whom the power of appointing or designeing for that turne is, doe come into the Chappell of the sayd *Hospitall*, and there before fower or more of the Brethren, do name him or her, whom in his conscience he findeth fittest. Which being done, the Maister or Vice-Maister shall conduct the person so named to the Chamber which is voyd, which he or she shall presently enioy, but not have any other Allowance of the Howse, till the end of one quarter of a yeare, the money that is saved being to be put into the Common Chest of the *Hospitall* to supply Reparations, Law-suites, and other Casualties. But after the end of three Monethes, the Brother or Sister designed shall in the Chappell of the Hospitall before the Maister, or Vice-Maister, first take the Oath of Allegeance or obedience to the *Kings* Maiestie, his heires and lawfull Successors according as by lawe it is prescribed and then this Oath ensuing. *I. A.B. from henceforth as long as I shall remaine a Member of this Hospitall of the Blessed Trinitie in Guildford, shall and will, by Gods assistance do my best endeauour to fulfill and keepe the Statuts and Ordinances of the same, so far forth as they concerne me. I shall be obedient to the Maister of the Hospitall in all honest and reasonable things. I shall not at any time willingly procure, or giue assent unto any indaungering, hurt or indomaging of the sayd Hospitall, either in the Estate, Hereditaments, or moueable goods thereof, but to my best power and skill, shall defend & set forward the welfaire and commoditie thereof whiles I live. So help me God in Jesus Christ.*

Heere I thinke fitt to adde this, That because it may fall out, that there be not men or women of Threescore yeares of age, and single persons in the towne to supply such places as are voyd, as in my owne life time I founde once by experience that there were not, I do give Licence, that in such Case, and no other, some aged maryed man or women be chosen, which is of qualitie and conditions other wayes agreeable to my Statutes. But in the Choice of such a person, I will have the consent of the Maior of Guildford, the Maister of the *Hospitall*, and the Parson of Trinity parish all concurring, because I will not haue this done but vpron necessitie. This man or woman shall have the weekely allowance of the *House*, and nothing else, and shall be called by the name of an Out-brother, or an Out-sister.

Appendix 2

Chap: 7:

Of the Service of God.

Among, or aboue all things, that such persons as remaine in this Hospitall are to do, it is the first to take care that God be served, who is the giver and continuer of all good things. The Maister therefore of the *Hospitall* shall so often as conveniently he can, reade some part of Divine Service, according to the booke of Common prayer, morning and Evening in the Chappell of the Hospitall to the Brethren and Sisters, & give God thankes for their Founder, and all other Gods benefits and blessings: And this to be every daye, except those hereafter mentioned. And if the Maister do not performe it himselfe, then the Vice maister (whom, I would alwaies have chosen such a one as can handsomely reade), or in his absence such a one of the Brothers as the Maister shall appoint, shall without grudgeing performe that office. There can noe man be too good to serve God.

On the Sabaoth dayes, Festivall dayes, wednesdayes, and Frydayes, at Morning and Evening prayers, and vpon Saterdayes at Evening prayer, all the Brethren and Sisters of the Hospitall, being at home and not sick (except the *Porter*, who is to tarry at home, to keepe the *House* in the absence of the rest) shall repair two and two in an orderly fashion to *Trinitie Church* which is neere vnto them, and there devoutly pray with the rest of the Congregation for the preservation of the Kings Maiestie, his Children and yssue when God sendeth them, as alsoe for the happines and prosperitie of his Kingdomes, and heare the word of God preached or read, and there be partakers of the Holy Sacrament of the Lords Supper, at the least thrice every yeare.

And to the end that all persons, who are able, may be present at prayers in the Chappell, or Parish Church, the Maister, or Vice-maister in his absence, shall weekly appoint one to note such as are absent from prayers, who shall dayly glue their names to the Maister, or in his absence to the Vice-maister; And if any without a sufficient cause, to be allowed by the Maister, or in his abscnce by the Vice maister, be not present, at prayers, hee or she shall for the first time forfeite an half penny; for the second a penny, and so for every time after in each moneth, to be abated and defalked from their allowance at the pay day happening next after such their default. Of theis forfeitures one third part is to be imployed to the Porter for that Moneth, and the other two to the Common Chest. But in case any one (without such cause as is aforesayd) shalbe found to have ben absent seaven times in one Moneth, he shall for the first time that he is found so offending, forfeit all his allowance of the Howse for one Forthnight, And for the second time hee or she shall have an Admonition solemnely given him or her by the Maister and Vice-maister, which shalbe entred into the Lidger Booke; But if after Three such Admonitions the same partie shalbe found againe to have offended in the same kinde, he or she shall then for a negligent and incorrigible person, be expelled from the *Hospitall*, never to be receaved there againe. For whie should any one, who will not serve God, be thought fitt to be in this Body.

After my departure out of this world I appoint that a Commemoration or Thankesgiving should be saide at prayer time dayly in the Chappel, for me as the Founder of this *Hospitall*, and for *Syr Nicholas Kempe, knight,* who was a Benefactor to this *House*. The substance of this *Commemoration* to be, That they thanke God for raising vp vnto them such a Founder and Benefactor, and do pray God, that they may use aright such benefitte as by their meanes have bene and are bestowed vpon them.

Chap: 8:

Of honest conversation.

Next after the Service of God, an honest and quiet Conversation is to be looked vnto, it being the Rule of the *Apostle*, That Christians should live godly, iustly, and soberly in this present worlde. I doe therefore wish, that the Brethren & Sisters of this Hospitall should live peaceably & quietly together, as having one heart, and one mynde, avoyding faction or banding and siding one against another, but studying to cherish, help, and comfort each other, especially in time of sicknes, striving with all goodnesse and humblenesse to beare one anothers burthen. I would have them by noe meanes to be haunters of Ale-howses or Tavernes for that ministreth occasion of Drunkennes, which is a vice odious to God, and good men, apt to bring on all kinde of sinne, and hath all the dayes of my life bene hatefull vnto mee.

Chap: 9:

What Crimes are to be avoyded, & uppon what Penalties

If any Brother or Sister shalbe Convicted of any kinde of Incontinency, Periurie, Forgery, obstinacy in Heresie, Sorcerie, or any sorte of Charming or Witchcraft, or of any Cryme punishable by losse of lyfe or lymme, or of eare, or shall be publickly set on the Pillory, or whipped for any offence by them committed, or shall obstinately refuse to frequent Divine Service by lawe established: Vppon Confession or Conviction heereof, before the Mayor of Guildford, the Maister of the *Hospitall*, and the Schoole-master of the Free-schoole, such Brother or Sister shall immediately by them be displaced and expelled out of the *House*, and shall never be receaved thither againe. And if any Brother or Sister shalbe a blasphemer of Gods holy name, an ordinary swearer, a Gamester at vnlawfull games, a Drunkard, or haunter of Tavernes and Ale-howses, a Brawler, fighter, contentious person, Scould, or sower of Discorde, and thereof shall be convicted by Confession or honest proofe before the Maister of the Hospitall, the Vice-Maister, and the Parson of Trinitie Church in Guilford, or any two of them, such offender shall, for the first time, have a solemne Admonition given him or her to be entred into the Lidger Booke; For the second time, shall forfeite all Allowance And Commoditie for one Moneth

Appendix 2

to the Common Chest, and shall have another solemne Admonition as before; And if he or shee offende in the like third time, that person shall be expelled the Hospitall for ever, by those Three or two of them which are last before named.

Chap: 10:
Of Residence within the Hospitall.

The eye of the Governour Doth best direct those things which are vnder his Charge, & therefore it is fitt that the Maister of the *Hospitall* bee present continually, if it may be. But because necessary business may call him sometimes away I allowe vnto him for his owne affaires (yf he have cause) two monethes in the yeare to be taken iontly or - severally at his discretion, so that alwayes when he goeth to lye two nights out of Towne, he doe enter it into the lidger booke. When he is abroad in businesse of the Hospitall, either for law-suites, or to visitt the possessionsof the Hospitall, I account him not absent. Yf his private necessities enforce his absence for more then two monethes, if he shall, before the greater parte of the Brethren at home, shew a reasonable cause, which shall be approved by them first, and then by the Maior of Guildford, I give vnto him one Moneth more, to be registred in the Lidger booke: But beyond this none shall have further power, saue the Archbishop of Canterbury for the time being, whom I beseech to be moderate herein, And so to provide, that by the absence of the Maister, the Hospitall be not suffered in any sorte to runne into Dilapidations of building or estate.

To each Brother and Sister I allow the space of two monethes absence in the yeare, if they haue cause to vse it, ioyntly or dividedly: But so, that they aske leaue of the Maister, or in his absence of the Vice-master, whom I would not have to be difficult in graunting them leave.

The time of their going forth shalbe recorded in the Lidger-booke. And to the ende that the Members of this Howse may not be much flitting abroade, but remaining at home, as it is fit for aged folkes, I appoint that no Brother or Sister, being absent for any whole weeke from the Hospitall, shall have any more than half their weekely allowance; and this not to be neither unlesse the Maister, and Vice-maister do give approbation therevnto. The Maister, Brethren & Sisters are not to lodge anywhere in Guildford, but in the Hospitall: And if any Brother or Sister, without a sufficient Cause to be allowed by the Maister, or in his absence by the Vice-maister, shall lodge out of the *House*, for the first time hee or shee shall forfeite two pence; for the second time Fower pence; for the third time Eightpence; for the fourth time, two shillings, and for the fifth time, the whole next monethes allowance: Theis forfeitures to be to the Common Chest. For the sixt time, such is to have a solemne Admonition to be entred in the Lidger booke. For the seaventh offence, in any one yeere, (which shalbe accounted to begin at the Feast of St Michaell) another Admonition is to be given & entred: But if within the same yeere he do transgresse againe, hee or shee shall then by the Maister and Vice-maister be expelled

Abbot's Hospital Guildford

the *Hospitall*. For that party who hath so much minde to be out of the *House*, whie should he be troubled so far as to be kept in it.

Chap: 11:
That noe strangirs lye within
the Hospetall.

As on the one side I have ben carefull that those of this *Societie* shall lodge within the House; so my Desire is as greate, that such as are strangers should not lye within the Hospitall. I have provided, that no maryed person may be of this Bodie, but experience in other places hath taught me, that Fathers and Mothers are not vnwilling to draw their Children and kinsfolkes vnto them, which will be both a burthen and disturbance to the *House*, and so will the receaving of other strangers be, besides the disorders tht cannot be foreseene; I do therefore Ordaine that no person whatsoever shall be lodged in the *Hospitall*, or continue there one whole night (saving the Maister, and the Brethren and Sisters) except they be necessary servants of the *House*. Onely I allow the Maister, or in his absence the Vice-maister in extremitie of sicknes, and not otherwise, to give leave to any Brother or Sister, to have one person of their kinred, or otherwise, to watch wth them, besides the help that they shall have from the rest of this Societie. But if any Brother or Sister do openly or secretly suffer any person to lye, or continue all the night, in their chambers, or any other place of the Hosritall, and be thereof convicted, hee or shee shall for the first time forfeite the whole allowance of a Moneth to the Common Chest, and for the second time, the benefitt that should come vnto him or her for a quarter of a yeare to be to the Common Chest as before; both theis to be entred with an Admonition into the Lidger-booke: But the partie, that the Third time transgresseth in this kinde, and is convicted thereof, before the Maister, Vice-maister, and Parson of Trinitie Church, shalbe by them for ever expelled out of the sayd Hospitall; And herein I require them to be strict and severe.

To the Maister of the *Hospitall* I give leave to intertain a servant or two for his necessary vses, but such as lie will be answerable for to the Societie. And because the Lodgeing provided for him hath convenient roomes, and sometimes ther may be extraordinary concourse unto the Towne as when the Court lyeth neere, or at the time of the Assize, or in some other cases which cannot be foreseene, I do permitt unto him to lodge either his frend, or some other person or persons of qualitie, so that it be not longer then for fouer or five nights. And the same libertie I allow to be used to my brother Sr Morris Abbott knight, or to any of his Children, or Childrens children, if they should have occasion to see Guildford. Provided always, that none of these bring any detriment or expence to the Hospitall.

Appendix 2

Chap: 12:

Care to be had of those that be sick.

It cannot be conceaved, but where aged people are, some are like diverse times to be sick, who are then to be attended and comforted; for in health each one can care for himself, but in sicknesse he must be helped by other. For the better performing of this, I appoint, first, that all the Sisters shall from time to time be carefull over the sick, as themselves would be wished to be helped by others in their extremities: where they are to remember, that as naturall sisters are loving to their Brothers and Sisters, especially in time of necessitie; So I would have theis to be kinde each to other, whom I as a common Father have incorporated into this Societie. And secondly, I ordaine, that yearely, the morrow after Michaelmas day, the Master shall appoint specially twoe of the Sisters whom he thinketh to be most fitt for tht purpose, to take upon them this particular charge, and Christian duetie. Theis shall be called the Releevers of the impotent; And when they have well and carefully performed that charge, at the end of the yeare, they shall have Six shillings and Eight pence a peece out of the Common Chest, as an augmentation of their allowance. But if any so appointed by the Maister shall refuse to take that Charge vppon them, the partie so refusing shall be debarred from receaving any allowance whatsoever for that yeare; And that which is saved from her shalbe put into the Common Chest of the Hospitall.

Chap: 13:

Of the Porter, and his Office.

There wilbe a necessitie of having a Porter to keepe the gates of the *House*, when the rest are gone to the parish Church, or otherwise vnto a Sermon. I do therefore Ordaine that the Five Junior Brethren shall in their turnes for the space of one moneth a peece supply this place, the Junior of all, first beginning, and so ascending upwards. And one the first day of every moneth, the Brother whose turne it is shall come unto the Maister, or in his absence to the Vice-maister, to receave his charge for tht place. His office shalbe to ring a Bell twise each morning and evening vnto prayers, the second ringing, to be one quarter of an houre after the first. He shall also in the Somer, betweene the Annunciation and Michaelmas, receave the keyes of the gates from the Maister or Vice-maister in the morning and open the foregate at seaven of the clock, and he shall shut it at eight of the clock in the evening during that time, and cary the keyes to the Maister, or in his absence to the Vice-maister, every night. And from the Feast of Michaelmas to the Annunciation, he shall open the gates about eight of the clock in the morning, and shut them at seaven a clock at night; and then carry the keyes to the Maister, or in his absence to the Vice-maister. The back gate shall not be opened, but when there is speciall use for Carriage, or otherwise, and when that is finished, it shall presently be shut againe.

Chap: 14:

Of the Reparations of the Hospitall.

I have caused this *House* to be substantially built, and with Gods blessing, together with the care of those who shall enioy it, the same may continue long without greate neede of Reparations. If any thing be amisse in the maine worke, I would have it presently amended, least neglect at the first bring on further decay. To this I ordaine, that yearely on the Monday next following the Feast of St John Baptist, the Maister, or Vice-maister in his absence, with three other of the Brethren whom he shall thinke aptest for that purpose, doe discreetely view the House in all buildings, the Sellars, Leades, together wth the Garden walls, and the house neere the garden, and where they finde cause, that, as soone as may be, they see it repayred; and if any tyle fall of, or any bricke be notedly missing in the building, or anything happen which can abide no delay for the mending, although it be in the winter time, I would have it repayred as soone as conveniently may be. And all things so done in the publicke structure, shall be at the expense of the Hospitall out of the Common Chest.

If in any private roome of the *Hospitall*, any glasse windowe be broken, or any other decay be by willfullnesse or negligence, that Brother or Sister, whose the roome is, shall at his or her charges, see it amended within the space of a Moneth, vpon warning given by the Maister, or Vice-maister; within which time, if it be not done, the person whose default it was, shall for every weeke forfeit Foure pence to goe to the Common Chest.

If the glasse of any publicke roome be broken, it shall first be enquired of, who was the cause thereof, and if it be found, the partye offending shall make it vp againe. And yf it cannot be discovered who it was, it shall bee repayred at the charge of the *Hospitall*.

But for the better preserving of all the glasse in the Howse, I do vtterly forbid the keeping of any Dogge within the Hospitall or precincts thereof, vpon paine, (to the partie offending) of forfeiting Five shillings to the Common Chest for every daye. And in this I require the Maister and Vice-maister vpon their oath to be very severe.

Chap: 15:

Of cleane keeping of the pub-
lick roomes.

It is a religious care that the house of God should be decently kept; and it is a seemely sight that publick places whereunto strangers may resort, do lye no otherwise then cleanly. I ordaine therefore, that on every Satterday in the afternoone the Chappell, and Hall be swept by one of the three Junior Sisters in their turnes, the latest commer into the *House* being first to begin, and so to the next in order. And if the Garden yeeld hearbes or flowers in the Somertime, they cannot be better imployed then to adorne these roomes. I do vtterly forbid any swine or other noisome beast to be kept within the precinct of the Hospitall or Back-side, because my desire is that both comelinesse and health should bee every way preserved.

Chap: 16:

In what worldly businesse the Brothers or Sisters may exercise themselves.

To the end that idlenesse may be avoyded, which is the mother of many sinnes, I doe not onely permitt, that any Brother or Sister who hath skill in any manuall Trade, do work in the same, either within the Hospitall or wthout, to gett some part of their living, but I do much commend them who shall imploy themselves that waye: But ever with this Caution, that their labouring within the *House* be not offensive by any greate noyse, ill savour or otherwise, to the rest of the Societie. I allowe also, that any *Brother* or *Sister* being able to exercise themselves in any honest labour of the body, may performe the same abroade, so that they lodge not out of the *Hospitall* without speciall leave of the *Maister*, or in his absence the Vice-maister, and that to be not above one night in the weeke. I doe forbid that any Brother or Sister should keepe any Ale-house or Vicualing howse within the Hospitall or without, vpon paine of loosing their places, *ipso facto*.

It shall not be lawfull for any Member of this Body, by themselves or other to begge or crave of any person within the Towne or elsewhere. If any be founde so to do, after two Admonitions given by the Maister, (which by vertue of his oath, after notice given, I charge him, to performe) he or she forthwith be expelled by the Maister; Yet if any person shall, without craving or asking, voluntarily give any Almes or benevolence, it shalbe lawfull for those that are present to receave it, and to put it into the Box prepared for that purpose, That so, when it cometh to any quantitie, it may be divided among the Brothers and Sisters equally; for I will not have the Maister to have any portion thereof. There shalbe two severall locks and keyes to this Boxe, the one to be kept by the Maister, the other by the senior Brother at home; And once in the quarter it shalbe opened in the presence of the most part of the Societie, to be distributed among all. *Provided* allwayes, That if anything be bestowed vpon any particular person, in respect of kinred sicknes or other impotency, that wholy shall goe to the partie on whome it is peculiarly and specially bestowed.

Chap: 17:

Of the House for the Evidences, and common Seale.

I have built a strong roome in the topp of the Tower over the gate, and although it be wthin the Maisters lodgeing, yet I would have three keyes to the doore thereof; The one to be kept by the Maister, the other by the Vice-Maister, the third by the senior Brother who is not Vice-maister. In this roome I appoint things of moment, which are not of dayly use, to be safely layd vp; And there shall be one Chest with three severall locks of sundry wardes and fashions, the keyes whereof shall be kept by the three above named. In this Chest shalbe kept the Common seale, a Copie of theis Statutes, and such stock of money as yearely remayneth after all Disbursements, and is to be reserved for Reparations, and other necessary vses.

I ordaine also, that there be in the same roome one other large Chest, wherein the Foundation of the Hospitall shall be kept, and all Evidences of Landes, sorted fitly into severall Boxes, which shall be superscribed with papers of direction according to the Landes, or parcells of the same. There shall also be put, all Rentalls, Surveyes, Terras, with buttailes and boundes, if any such be; Counter-paines of Leases, Court-Rowles and yearely Accounts; And to this Chest there shalbe also three several locks and keyes to be kept, by the Maister one, by the most Aunciant Brother the second, and the third by one other of the Brethren, who, from yeare to yeare the morrow after Michaelmas day, shalbe chosen by the maior parte of the Brethren of the *Hospitall*.

I ordaine, that noe parcell of Evidence shall at any time be taken forth thence, but vpon speciall cause, and then also not to be longer kept from thence, then necessary occasion for the vse thereof shall require.

There shall also remaine in the said Chest, a paper booke wherein shalbe entred the parcels of all Evidences from time to time taken forth, the day and yeare when, and to whose hands it was delivered, and for how long time as is to be presupposed; And the day and yeare also shall be entred, when and by whom such pcells of Evidence is delivered in againe.

Chap: 18.

Of the Books and Register of the Hospital.

In such a roome of the Maisters lodgeing as I shall appoint, there shall be a faire Lidger Booke kept with lock and keye, wherein by the Maister or Vice-Maister shalbe entred and Registered, the names, age, qualitie and times of admittance of every Maister, Brother and Sister, as also the times of their remoovings or deathes. There shall also be one other faire Lidger Booke, wherein shall be entred the Copies of all Leases or other Grauntes that be presently in *Esse* or hereafter shalbe made by the sayd Hospitall, And there shalbe a third Lidger Booke, wherein shall be Entred such things as are given unto them of any moment, and by whom; And the Inventory of all their moveables; And also all other matters that be of weight, and may be fitt by Record to be continued to posteritie; But especially such Admonitions as are given to offenders, according to theis Statutes.

Chap: 19:

*How their Lands shalbe demised, &
with what Covenants &E, How
their Woods are to be kept , And
both wood & Lands surveyed.*

 The Lande and howses wch I give to the Hospitall, are intended by me to be for the good thereof, and that in perpetuitie, if God so be pleased. I doe therefore in this Chapter lay downe such Conditions as are fitt to be observed in their Demises; as first: That no Lease or any other Graunt shalbe made of any landes Tenementes or Hereditamentes belonging to this Hospitall, vnles the Maister, Vice maister, and besides them, the greater Part of the Brethren do yeeld their consentes therevnto; Nor vnlesse the full accustomed yearely Rent thereof, according as I do leave it, be therevpon reserved and payable quarterly or at least half yearely, at or within the said Hospitall. And such Lease or graunt shall not be above Twentie and one yeares from the making of the same by the Hospitall, And with Reservation of all Timber trees. And in the sayd Lease shalbe conteyned the true and Perfect parcells and quantity of Landes by common estimation, with the Buttalls and boundals thereof, if conveniently it may be. Secondly ther shalbe in every such Lease or grante a *Proviso* conteyned, That the Farmor or Tenant shall pay the Rent at the *Hospitall* wthin Twentie dayes next ensuing any one Rent day limited for payment thereof, without any Demaund to be made. Furthermore in each Lease or grant to be made, Covenantes of this effect shall be. First, that the Lessee at his owne Cost shall not onely repayre, and if neede be, reedifie all Edifices thereupon; and so well reedifyed and repaired shall leave them at the end of the terme, But shall also from time to time, hedge, fence ditch and scowre the grounds according to the usual course of husbandry of the Countrey where the sayd lands do lye. Secondly, that the sayd Lessee shall beare, pay and discharge, or save harmeles the sayd *Hospitall* of & from all charges ordinary and extraordinary going out or to be payed by reason of the Lands Demised, or any part thereof. Lastly, that the Lessee, betwixt every eight and ninth years of the said Terme, shall make or cause to be made and written faire in parchment, and deliver up to the Maister at the *Hospitall*, a true and perfect Terrar, conteyning the name & quantity, (by estimation) of every parcell of grounde Demised, the manner of the situation and lying of the same towards other lands, and the names of the present owners of the lands which are of any side abutting vpon the groundes Demised.

 I doe ordaine and appoint, that the sayd Hospitall, vpon any Reservation or otherwise, shall not increase their Rent or Revenewes of those Landes I shall give vnto them, to any higher or greater proportion, then as the Rents thereof now are and according to that rate they are now lett for. Vnlesse it fall out that vpon necessitie, which cannot be avoyded, some one of their Farmes do diminish in their Rents wch I ordaine shall be moderately supplyed by raysing somewhat vpon some other Farme which may well beare it. For I desire that, my *Hospitall* should keepe up the Rent, wherwth all I do endow it. But I do

Abbot's Hospital Guildford

charge the Consciences of the Maister and Brethren, that they bee very wary and carefull before they make any such alteration.

I do also ordaine, that in Renuing and letting of Leases, the Present Farmors and Tenantes be always preferred, doing reasonably for the benefitt of the *Hospitall* as other men will doe: And among the rest I would have those especially favoured, who have their Leases from myselfe, or by my direction.

And also I do ordaine and appoint tht such money as they shall raise, or make vppon the fines of Leases, shalbe divided into two parts, the one moytie to be distributed betweene the Maister, Brethren and Sisters equally, saving that the Maister shall have a double portion. The other moytie to be put into the common Treasury, for the bearing of publicke burthens, as suites of lawe, Reparations, or the like. For the Vnderwoodes if they be not in my tyme leased out, I would have to be cutt in due season, and yearely, looke what profitt is made thereof, that it should be accounted as part of their Revenewe, and goe to the common charges of the *House*. But no Tymber trees to be sould, but vpon greate necessitie, or apparant shew of decay, and the money arysing thereof to be put into the common Treasury, not to be expended but vpon greate occasions.

Chap: 20:

By whom the Revenewes of the Hospitall are to be Receaued, and disbursed.

The Revenewes and Rents of the Howse shalbe receaved in the Hospitall, by the Maister, Vice-maister, and the other Clavigers or key-keepers, And they shall give their Acquittance for it. If either of theis places be voyd, or any of them be out of towne, or so sick, that they cannot be present at this Receite, Then in their steede, shall be called, the next two Brothers in auncientry that are able to stirr abroade, they taking vnto them (if neither of them can write) some of the Brethren that can write, or some other honest person who is able to write; and presently vpon receite of the Rent, an Entry shalbe made thereof into the Lidger booke; And then immediately shall the money be layd vp in the Common Chest, there to remaine till there be occasion, for paymentes, to take it cut againe.

When any Quarter is ended, tile next day if be not Sunday, or if it be so, then the next day following; the Clavigers or Chest-keepers shall assemble in the Maister's lodgeing, and taking forth of the common Chest so much money onely as is to be disbursed, they shall pay vnto each Brother and Sister their severall due Allowances, a note of the Receite thereof being presently made in the Lidger-booke. And if any be sick or absent, it shalbe payd to such a Brother as hee or shee shall make their Attorney. And then shall the Maister also receaue his allowance.

Appendix 2

If, besides the Quarterly wages or allowance, there happen any occasion for Disbursement of money otherwise, as for Reparations, or suits in Lawe, or some such like thing, this shall be entred into the Lidger Booke, the day being named and the occasion, and in whose presence, and to whom it was delivered, together with his hand or marke that receaved it.

Chap: 21:
Of Accoumpts to be made for the
whole yeare.

There is nothing that maketh any *Corporation* so to florish, as good husbandry, and diligent looking to the state thereof; And if I your Founder in the course of my life had not ben provident that way, how should I haue bene able to builde this House, and endow it with possessions; And therefore I do appoint that on the Nine and Twentith of October (which was the day whereon I was borne) yearely, the Maister, Vice-master, Clavigers, and two other of tile Brothers which are most auncient, and be in no office, or key-keepers, shall meete together in the Maisters lodgeing, end there shall well examine what Rentes or money of the Common stock hath ben receaved that yeare; As also what hath ben spent every way; and if they have exceeded in expence (which god forbid) they shalbe carefull to sett some course, that in the yeare to come it be more frugally and thriftily carryed. And if there by any surplusage of money beyond the expences for the yeare past which ended at Michaelmas, they shall carry that vp to be put in the common Chest: And they shall alwayes, at the time of their Accoumpte, sett downe in the lidger-booke, what the stocke of money is which remayneth over and aboue the expences of the yeare. Theis Accoumptes I ordaine to be ended before *Alhalowne* day yearely. If the nine and twentith day of October fall on the Sonday, then the Accoumptes shall begin the morrow after.

When the Accoumptes are ended, the Maister or Vice-maister shall in the Hall upon Allhalowne day, declare to all the Brothers and Sisters, what the whole Somme of the Receiptes was the yeare past, what also was the Somme of that which hath ben expended, what remayned in Stock of the Howse, the yeare twelue moneth before, and what is the remainder this present yeare, that all of them may praise the diligence and faithfulnesse of those that manage the money, or disprayse it, if there be cause.

If there be founde to be any Arrerages in any of the Accountantes handes, the same shal either presently be payd, or, within three dayes at the furthest, be delivered to the Clavigers, to be layd vp in the Common Chest, vpon payne of losse of the next monethes allowance of him that shalbe so behinde; But if after the sayd three dayes be expired the whole Arrerages shall not be payd within Thirtie dayes, that partie in whom the default is, shall, *ipso facto*, loose his place, and be sued in lawe for the Arrerages remayning.

Abbot's Hospital Guildford

I do ordaine, that none of the money belonging to the common Chest, shall, vpon paine of periurie in all those that give consent therevnto, be lent out to any person whatsoever, either within the *Hospitall*, or without; For no particular mans case is to be preferred before the publick good of the *Howse*, before order, and the will of mee the Founder.

Chap: 22:

Of the Reading of the Statutes

That all the Members of this Hospitall, may vnderstand my minde for their good governement, and each of them knowe their Duetie one to another; I do ordaine and appoint, that in the Chappell on the wednesday in Easter weeke yearely, the Maister, or Vice-maister, or some one of the Brethren who can reade most distinctly, and shall, by the Maister, or in his absence by the Vice-Maister, be appointed therevnto, shall reade over the whole booke of theis Statutes to the whole Societie; And if they be too long to be read vppon one day, I allow more times, so that the whole be read through by the Satterday of that weeke. If any Brother or Sister be absent at theis times without a sufficient cause allowed by the Maister, or Vice-maister, hee or shee shall forfeite Twelve pence for every time; And if any refuse to reade being appointed, he shall forfeit for every time of refusing, Five shillings, those Sommes to goe to the Common Chest.

Chap: 23:

How the Maister, if he transgress is to bee Censured.

I do Ordaine, That if the Maister of my Hospitall, shall be found to be negligent in performing the Duetie and Charge which is imposed vpon him by theis Ordinances, then vpon notice thereof given to the Archbishop of Canterbury for the time being, such punishment shall be inflicted vppon him, as the said Lo: Archbishop in his Discretion shall thinke convenient.

Chap: 24:

Of the Chambers in the Hospitall.

I appoint, and my will is, That the Maisters lodgeing shalbe reserved for my selfe, during my life, if I see cause to vse it; And then, if I do make vse of it, the Maister for the tyme being, shall have his lodgeing in the North-west part of the *Hospitall*; yet so, that those to whom it apperteyneth to go into the Evidence house, or to doe other businnesse designed in these Statutes, shall have accesse at all convenient times into the Lodgeing reserved for myself. My Executor also shall have the vse of my lodgeings for himself if he will, for one yeare after my decease. *Provided*, that he designe it not over to any other, nor place any therein, vnlesse it be some Member of my *Hospitall*. The other Chambers shalbe assigned to the Brothers and Sisters of the *Hospitall*, and as any of them shall fall voyd, the next successor shall come into the sayd Roome. I do onely except the corner Chamber on the South-west side, which being a double Chamber, I assigne to such a person as hath borne office in the Towne if any such be, to be bestowed by myself for my life time, and afterwards at the Discretion of the Maister.

Chap: 25:

Of the Visitor of the Hospitall.

I doe reserve vnto my selfe, during my life, power to abrogate, adde vnto, change or alter these Ordinances, And to place or displace any Member thereof with cause or without cause to be rendred thereof to any other; to lett Leases, and wholy to governe the same as I shall see reason, and this to be during my naturall life, without any other persons intermedling therein. And after my Decease, I ordaine and appoint the Lord Archbishop of Canterbury from tyme to tyme to be the *Visitors* of the said Hospitall, whom I do beseech in the bowells of *Jesus Christ*, to have a fatherly and compassionate care of the good estate thereof, as alsoe of the poore Members of the same. The power of the Archbishop shall be, by himself, or others whom he shall appoint, to interpret any doubt arysing out of theis Ordinances and Statutes, and to punish, Censure, and remoove any Member thereof convicted according to these Ordinances by me sett downe.

The sayd Archbishop also from time to time shall have authoritie by himself, or other whom he shall appoint, to Visite this *Hospitall*, and the Members thereof, to Compose their Controversies, to direct and advise them, as also to enquire of the publick State of the *House*, and of the private behaviour of all persons in the same; And if other men, to whom I have given any Charge or power in Nomination of pursons into the Hospitall, or of remooving them out of it, or any other matter whatsoever, do not their Dueties according to these Statutes, That then the said Lo: Archbishop by himself, or other, shall see it reformed, for which fatherly care I do not doubt, but God will returne many blessings vppon him.

Chap: 26:

*Of such Allowances as are to be made
to the Maister, and members
of this Hospitall.*

The benefite that the Maister is to reape by the Hospitall shall be Twenty pounds in money to be receaved by equall portions at the Foure Quarters in the yeare, the Lodgeing assigned vnto him; a Livery gowne, and a double portion of such Dividend in money as is to arise by Fynes taken for renewing of Leases when it shall fall out. I appoint to every Brother and Sister Two shillings six pence, to be weekly payd vnto them, their Chamber, and their Livery, besides such money as may arise by letting of Leases hereafter, and from the poore mens Boxe.

And Concerning Gownes, this I doe ordaine, That once in two yeeres against Allhalownetide, there be bought Cloth good and strong, of price about Nine or Ten shillings the London yarde, out of the which the Maister shall have the allowance fitt for a large Gowne, and each Brother and Sister so much as will make vnto them a reasonable gowne according to the tallnesse or stature of the partie that is to weare it, that in these gownes they may go to the *Trinity Church* or other place where the Sermon is to be. The Badges are to be accounted to belong to the *Hospitall*, and must descend to those that come in from time to time. And if any dye, his or her gowne is to be left to the vse of those who shall succeede, that the Hospitall be not drivento buy Liveries but at the time appointed. Notwithstanding when new Gownes are bought and made, it shalbe at the will of every one to cut out their olde, or to dispose of them at their pleasure. The Maister is to take care of these things, as also of buying sea-cole, or Char-cole every yeere that may serve for the publicke vse, betweene Alhalowne tide, and our Lady day in Lent. If this be got in, in the Somer time, it will be the cheaper, because the wayes are fairer. When the wood that I bought of Bromfeld shall bee growne fitt, I appoint that such fewel as may be taken of it, be vsed without spoile in the Cutting, and this will save some money, which is otherwise to be layd out.

I do appoint that yeerely on Christmas day there bee expended Ten shillings among the Company publikely in the Hall, in remembrance of the Birth of our Saviour Christ. And the like summe on Easter day, as also upon Whit sonday, that the Maister, Brethren and Sisters may with thankes to God lovingly rejoyce together. And I appoint other ten shillings to be bestowed vpon the Nine and twentith of October yeerely, in Commemoration of the birth day of their Founder.

Chap: 27:

*Touching the Manufacture to
bee sett vp.*

In the procuring of my Letters of Mortmaine, one principall matter intended by me, was to sett vp some Manufacture in the Towne of *Guilford*, that young people might be set on worke, and that, by trading, that place might flourish as heretofore it hath done.

I have taken order, if God do blesse it, for land of one hundred poundes by the yeere to be purchased for that purpose. And when it shall bee done, I intreatre the Maior of *Guildford* & his Brethren solemnely to meete once or more times in the yeere, and to call vnto them such wise and disereete persons as they shall thinke fitt, to advise whereuppon this Imployment may best be fastened, as on Hempe, knitting of stockings, or wastcotes, or any other lawdable Trade that may bee for the good of the Common wealth, or that Corporation in particular.

And I do pray these persons which shall so meete, to thinke vpon Orders to be sett in writing for the digesting of the worke, and how once at the least in the yeere, there may be an Account taken how this Manufacture doth prosper, and what is from time to time to bee altered, added, or amended in the Proiect. If God send mee life I shall think vpon the advauncing and establishing of this my intendement, which I do earnestly desire, that a beginning may be given to the worke.

For the erecting and continuing of this Manufacture, I do appoint the Lande at *Charlewood* bought of one Polesden, which is lett for Fourty pounds yeerely wch rent I order to be applied onely to that purpose. And in the like manner I appoint the Lande at Burstow bought of Mr *Bishe* and being rented at Three score poundes by the yeare, to be imployed solely for this Manufacture. So that I do ordaine that this hundred pounds by the yeare shall not be mingled wth any other money of my *Hospitall*, but the rent thereof to be put into a Chest by it selfe, and all accounts appertayning therevnto to be kept and reserved by themselves. I appoint that vpon this Chest be written and fastened in paper, *The Chest for the Manufacture*, and three locks and keyes shall be thereunto, which keyes shalbe kept by the Maister, Vice maister, and the seniour keyekeeper. And in this Chest shall always bee a greate Lidger booke, wherein shalbee sett downe what mony for the Manufacture is receaved in, and what is layd out, and the Accounts at the end of the yeare shall be there kept that it may be seene how the benefitt by the trade increaseth or decreaseth.

I do not tye them that haue charge of this worke to any one certain trade, but give them power at the end of the yeare (wch I wishe to be vpon the tenth or eleventh of November,) to alter it, if they finde reason for the same. But I appoint that this alteration shall be vpon greate deliberation and good grounde, least by too much shifting all come to nothing.

I do ordaine, that some discreete man who dwelleth in the towne of Guildford, and writeth a faire hande, be chosen for a Clarke, to write downe things necessary for the stablishing of this worke; And for this I appoint him to have twentie shillings yearely at or vppon the tenth of November: And if the worke do prosper it shall be in the power of the Overseers for this worke, to better his paye, so that it do not exceede twentie shillings more in any one yeare.

Chap: 28:

*The proportion of the Rents of the
Hospitall, & the Allowances out of them.*

The mentioning of the Clerks fee for the Manufacture, doth put me in minde to sett downe an establishment of the Revenew for my Hospitall, and the Expences which must issue out of the same. The Land then that I have endowed it withall (the Rents whereof I would never have increased or decreased, if it may be) are these.

The Lande at Merrow, which was bought of Mr Har=
=Ward, by the yeare / ──────── Fowre score poundes.
The land at Meredin, bought of Mr Goodwin, by the
yeare / ──────────────────── Fourtie Pounds.
The Lande at Ewerst, bought of Thomas Hill, by the
yeare / ────────── Twentie Seaven pounds ten shillings.
The lande at Horsham, bought of Constable, by the
yeare / ─────────────────── Fourtie Pounds.
The woodlande bought of Bromfielde, by the
yeare / ───────────── Twelve Pounds ten shillings.
In the whole some this amounteth to by the yeare,
/ ─────────────────────────── Two hundred Poundes.

Out of the Receits, I do make this proportion
of yearely Allowances.
To the Maister of the Hospitall by the yeare / ──────── Twentie
poundes.
To Twentie poore Brothers and Sisters / ────────── Two shil=
=lings six pence a peece by the weeke, which in the
yeare amounteth to / ────────── One hundred & thirty pounds.
To the Vice-maister yeerely / ───────── Thirteene shillings
Fowre pence.
To the two Releevers of the Impotent / ───────── Thirteene
shillings fowre pence.
For fowre Gaudy dayes / ──────────────── Fourty shillings.
For the Clerke to Record thinges, and for reading
the Statutes yearely / ────────── Twentie shillings.
To the Parson of *Trinitie Church* yearely / ─────────── Thirtie
shillings.
The totall of all which expence yearely amounteth
to / ────────── One hundred fiftie five poundes, sixteene shil=
=lings eight pence.

There remayneth then over and above yeerely, the somme of Fourty foure pounds three shill: foure pence, which I ordaine to this vse. That once in two yeeres there should

Appendix 2

be bought Three score yardes of Cloth London measure, to make new gownes for the Maister, Brothers and Sisters, which Cloth may be strong good Cloth, and may arise in the whole to about Thirtie poundes, whereof Fifteene poundes was saved the yeere before, and fifteene poundes to be taken out of the rent of that yeere when the Gownes are bought.

Out of the rest of the surplusage of the Revenew, I appoint fewell to be bought yeerely, which is to be burnt in Common, for the reliefe of the poore Brothers & Sisters from Alhalowne tide to Easter, which may amount to about

If any wood or Coale be had, towards this, out of the lande bought of Bromfeeld, it may save so much money otherwise. But I do order, that the said land of Bromfields be so disposed of, that it may yeeld Rent or wood or coale to the proportion before sett downe by mee, that the *Hospitall* may honestly enjoy that which I have payd for.

When all these expences we yssued forth, there will be a convenient surplusage remayning yeerely for the stock of the House, to beare Law suites, Reparations, or other publicke charge of the *Hospitall*, which wilbe the more increased by such money as will arise out of that quarters pay wch is forborne vppon the coming in of every Brother & Sister at the first. And this Stock I ordaine to be so carefully kept for the publicke, that if the Maister or any Brother shall take out for any private imployment the value of one shilling or vpward, vpon any colour, I appoint, that being convicted thereof before the Archbishop of Canterbury, he shall presently, by the said Lo: Archbishop be expelled the Howse.

When this Stock ariseth to an Hundred poundes, I would have that Summe carefully kept in golde against time of extremitie, and none of it to be taken out without greate cause; and yett then vpon the first opportunitie to bee made vp againe, because I hold it convenient that this my foundation should not be without one Hundred pounds lying by against any greate neede; which I hold fitt should be kept as a secret of the howse, and not be reveiled by the Maister, or any Brother of the Howse to any stranger whatsoever The rest which is above this Hundred poundes, is to be as a running Stock safely kept, but vpon necessary occasions money to be taken out for the publicke vse of the *Hospitall* from time to time.

Chap: 29:

The Explanation of a Clause in the second Chapter of these Statuts.

It was in the yeare of our Lord *1619* that I first intended the building of this *Hospitall*. And then minding the good of the Towne of Guildford in laying downe the persons that should be capable of places in my Foundation, I declared that for such as were borne, or did dwell twentie yeares in Guildford, I would have Guildford to be vnderstood that alone which was vnder the governement of the Maior of that towne, and not otherwise. Wherein, when I did straighten the extent of the place, it was not out of want of Charitie to other, but to increase my favour to the Inhabitantes there, in desiring that there should be provision for them and somewhat to spare, if God were so pleased.

Now since that time, before I had quite established my works, I do heare that the Maior and his Brethren have endeavoured toenlarge their Iurisdiction, and have gone about to drawe vnder theire governement some places adioyning, as if they were hereafter to be Members of that Corporation, and consequently capable of such benefittes as may arise by the government of that Towne. I will not dispute whether this endevour be well or no, for I have nothing to do with it: but for avoyding of controversie in future times, I do hereby declare, that my setled purpose and meaning is, that from henceforth I appoint none to be capable of my *Hospitall* which was not borne or lived not twenty yeares in Guildford, the towne of Guildford being taken as it was in the yeere *1620*, and not according to any addition that hath ben made since, or may be hereafter.

Whereof, if I should be demaunded a reason, it were a sufficient aunswere, to aske as it is in the Gospell, *May I not do what I will with mine owne?* But I have many other causes and reasons to declare as I now do. As first, I keepe myselfe to my first purpose and intention. Secondly it was the good of Guildford, old Guildford as it was when I was borne, and my Parentes lived in it, that I did seeke, which I did knowe would be the greater to the poore of that place, when it was restrayned within it selfe, and not communicated to any other. Thirdly, it is well knowne that I was borne in the parish of *St Nicholas* in that towne, vnto which parishe are belonging many howses in and about Katherine Hill, vnto whom notwithstanding I did not enlarge my benevolence, because they were not vnder the governement of the Maior, and my desire was and is, to keepe my Charitie wthin boundes, that after my death things may goe on quietly and there be no variance or controversie. Now if I have thus restrained the place where I was borne, it shall not be well if any other neighboures shall murmure thereat, or be discontented therewithall. I do therefore charge the Maister and Brethren of the Hospitall that they never give way to any importunitie that may or doth crosse this my explanation and Declaration.

These Statutes were finished & deliuered to be the Ordinances, whereby the Hospitall of the blessed Trinitie in Guilford is to be gouerned.

August: 17. 1629	G. Cant:
In the presence of	
Morris Abott	Maurice Abbott
Ri: Brigham	Walt: Dobson

Appendix 3

THE VICTORIAN STATUTES

22nd and 23rd Victoria, cap. 32.

An Act for confirming a Scheme of the Charity Commissioners, for "The Hospital of the Blessed Trinity," at *Guildford*, in the County of *Surrey*, and its subsidiary Endowments, with certain Alterations. [11th *July*, 1861.]

WHEREAS the Charity Commissioners for *England* and *Wales* in their Report to Her Majesty of their proceedings during the Year One thousand eight hundred and sixty, have reported that they have provisionally approved and certified, among other Schemes for the Application and Management of Charities, a Scheme for "The Hospital of the Blessed Trinity" at *Guildford* in the County of *Surrey*, and its subsidiary Endowments, and such Scheme is set out in the Appendix to their said Report: And whereas it is expedient that the said Scheme, as the same is set out in the Schedule to this Act, should be confirmed: Be it enacted by the Queen's most excellent Majesty, by and with the Advice and Consent of the Lords Spiritual and Temporal, and Commons, in this present Parliament assembled, and by the Authority of the same, as follows:

8th Report dated 26th February, 1861.

1. The said Scheme shall be confirmed and take effect.

Scheme in Schedule confirmed.

Abbot's Hospital Guildford

SCHEDULE.

SCHEME for the Application and Management of the CHARITY called "THE HOSPITAL of the BLESSED TRINITY," at GUILDFORD, in the COUNTY of SURREY, and its subsidiary Endowments.

1. The existing incorporation of the Master, Brethren, and Sisters of the Hospital of the Holy Trinity in Guildford, by that or any other name, shall be dissolved.

The Charity shall be under the management of thirteen Governors, to be called "The Governors of Trinity Hospital at Guildford," and to consist of nine official Governors, viz,:-

> The Mayor of Guildford;
> The Rector of the parishes of Holy Trinity and Saint Mary in Guildford;
> The Rector of the parish of Saint Nicholas in Guildford;
> The Rector of Stoke-next-Guildford;
> The Master of the Grammar School in Guildford respectively for the time being; and
> The two senior Aldermen and two senior Town Councillors of Guildford respectively for the time being, who shall respectively be members of the Church of England;

and of four non-official Governors, being fit and proper persons, resident in the town of Guildford, or within the distance of seven miles therefrom, who shall be appointed in the first instance by the Board of Charity Commissioners for England and Wales, with the concurrence of the Archbishop of Canterbury, within three months next after the establishment of this scheme.

2. The office of a non-official Governor shall be vacated by his resignation, or bankruptcy or insolvency, or his ceasing to reside within the limit aforesaid, or his refusal or incapacity to act, or omission for a period of two consecutive years to attend any meeting of the Governors; and as soon as conveniently may be after the occurrence of any vacancy among the non-official Governors from any of the causes aforesaid, or by the death or any such Governor, the remaining Governors for the time being shall select some fit person resident within the limit aforesaid to fill such vacancy, so as to keep up the full number of four non-official Governors: provided that every such election shall be forthwith notified by the Governors to the Charity Commissioners for England and Wales, and to the Archbishop of Canterbury; and the appointment of the new Governor shall not be complete until the same shall have been approved by the said Commissioners and the Archbishop; and provided also, that during any vacancy among the Governors the remaining Governors shall be competent to exercise all the authorities hereby vested in the Governors for the time being.

Appendix 3

3. All the real estate, of whatsoever tenure, and rights and privileges, belonging to or held in trust for the Charity (subject to the subsisting leases thereof, and the full benefit of all subsisting covenants, conditions, and securities made or reserved to the master and brethren of the said hospital, or to any person or persons in trust for them, or for the benefit of the Charity), and all the personal estate belonging thereto, and the right to sue for and recover all choses in action recoverable for the benefit thereof, shall be immediately vested in the said Governors hereby appointed, and shall from time to time vest and continue vested in the Governors of the said hospital for the time being, for the purposes and according to the provisions of this scheme, without any conveyance, assignment, or assurance; and the right to sue upon and enforce all covenants, conditions, or securities made or reserved to the said master and brethren before their dissolution, or to or with any preceding Governors of the said Charity, shall be exerciseable by them, in the name of the Governors of the said hospital for the time being, as fully and effectually as the same right might be exercised by such master and brethren if not dissolved, or by such preceding Governors, if still retaining their office; and in the same manner all contracts and liabilities of the said master and brethren, or of any preceding Governors for the time being of the said Charity, may be enforced against the Governors thereof for the time being, to the extent of the property or assets of the Charity, but not against their private estates.

4. The sum of £2,909 17s., part of the sum of £3,904 15s. 6d. new 3 per cent. annuities, now standing in the names of the Master and Brethren of the Hospital of the Blessed Trinity in Guildford, and all or any other sums of stock belonging to or held in trust for the benefit of the said hospital or the inmates thereof, including the sum of £2,000, 3l. per cent. consolidated annuities, arising from Molineux's Gift, and now standing in the names of Benjamin Kingston Finnimore, Charles Edward Mangles, Edmund Nicholls, and Joseph Weale, shall be transferred into the name of the Official Trustees of Charitable Funds in trust for the said hospital, and shall constitute part of the general endowment of the hospital. The sum of £994 18s. 6d., the remaining part of the said sum of £3,904 15s. 6d., new 3l. per cent. annuities, shall be transferred into the name of the Official Trustees aforesaid, in trust for Archbishop Abbot's School in Guildford.

5. The real estate and hereditaments constituting the Joint endowment of the said hospital and the aforesaid Archbishop Abbot's School (two-thirds of the rents whereof are payable to the hospital, and the remaining one-third to the Trustees of the said school), shall be divided in those proportions between the said hospital and school by a valuer to be appointed for the purpose by the said Board, who shall be at liberty to assign to such valuer such remuneration as to them shall seem fit, to be paid in the like proportions out of the funds of the hospital and school respectively, and on the execution by such valuer of his award or instrument of partition the respective shares of the hospital and the school in such estate and hereditaments shall vest in the said Governors and Trustees respectively, to be held by them in severalty for the purposes of the respective Charities.

Abbot's Hospital Guildford

6. The Governors shall, as soon as conveniently may be after the establishment of this scheme, subject to the approval of the said Board, make suitable regulations for the conduct and management of all matters connected with the administration of the Charity and its property, and may from time to time, with the like approval, vary such regulations; and all such regulations shall be binding upon all persons interested; provided that no regulation be so made which is at variance with any of the provisions of this scheme.

7. The Governors shall, out of the annual income of the Charity, pay the yearly sum of £1 10*s.* to the rector of the aforesaid parish of Holy Trinity in Guildford, and defray or provide for the expense of repairing and keeping insured the hospital and other buildings belonging to the Charity, and the necessary current outgoings and expenses of managing the said Charity.

8. The establishment of the hospital shall in future consist of a master and twenty brethren and sisters.

The master shall be a single person of good character, not less than 50 years old at the time of his appointment, and a native of Guildford, or resident there for a period of at least 20 years.

The brethren and sisters shall be respectively poor single persons of good character, not less than 60 years old at the time of appointment, natives of the ancient borough of Guildford, or resident there for a period of at least 20 years; provided that if and so often as there shall not be any duly qualified candidate from the said ancient borough, candidates from the municipal borough of Guildford, being otherwise duly qualified as directed by this scheme, shall be eligible for appointment. No person shall be eligible for any of the said appointments who is a drunkard or lunatic, or has any infectious or contagious disease, or who shall be in receipt of relief from any parochial or other rate for the relief of the poor, or who shall have received such relief at any time within the three next preceding years; and in the selection of candidates those persons are to be preferred who, being otherwise properly qualified, shall have borne office or been traders in the said borough of Guildford. The brethren and sisters shall in general be in the proportion of twelve brethren to eight sisters, with power, nevertheless, for the Governors to relax this rule under special circumstances as they may find expedient.

9. Upon the occurrence of any vacancy in the office of master, a meeting of the Governors shall be held, at which some proper person shall be appointed by the Governors to fill the vacancy; provided that no appointment of a master shall be made until the expiration of six weeks after the vacancy in the office has occurred, and that every such appointment be forthwith notified by the Governors to the Archbishop of Canterbury for his approval, without which approval the appointment shall not be complete or valid.

10. All applications for admission as inmates shall be made in writing to the master, and shall be entered by the master in a register specifying the date, and the name, age, residence, description, and qualifications of every applicant. The master shall also keep a register of all inmates admitted to the hospital, in which register shall be entered the

Appendix 3

date of every admission, and the particulars of the qualifications of each person admitted and the date and mode of occurrence of every vacancy,

11. All appointments of inmates shall be made by the Governors at some meeting of their body, and the persons to be so appointed shall be selected by the Governors from the register of applicants, and (except in such special or urgent cases as may be considered by the Governors to require the relaxation of this rule) no appointment of any inmate shall be made until after the expiration of one calendar month at the least from the date of his or her application for admission. In making the appointments preference shall in all cases be given by the Governors, as far as possible, to the most deserving candidates, qualified as aforesaid, regard being had to the age, personal character, and the circumstances and necessities of each candidate.

12. The master shall receive a yearly salary of £70, to be paid to him by the Governors half-yearly out of the income of the Charity, and an allowance of £5 annually for coals, and shall occupy such rooms within the hospital as may from time to time be assigned by the Governors for his use. The Governors, however, with the consent in writing of the Archbishop of Canterbury, and with the sanction of the Charity Commissioners, may from time to time vary the amount of the stipend and allowance to be paid to the master.

13. The Governors shall pay to each of the brethren and sisters respectively such weekly or other stipends or allowances, not exceeding the rate of 8*s*. per week, as the income and resources of the Charity will from time to time admit; provided that if the available income of the Charity at any time will not admit of the payment of a stipend at the rate of 5*s*. per week to each brother and sister the Governors shall be at liberty, with the consent of the Charity Commissioners, to suspend the appointment of the full number of inmates, so that such inmate may receive a stipend amounting to that weekly rate at the least.

The Governors shall also be at liberty to make reasonable allowances of coal or other necessaries to each of the brethren and sisters, to be provided out of the income of the Charity in addition to their pecuniary stipends, whenever such income shall be sufficient for the purpose.

14. The salary of the master and the weekly stipend of each brother and sister hereafter to be elected shall commence from the day of his or her admission to the hospital; but the Governors shall be at liberty, if they so think fit, to set apart any proportion, not exceeding one half of such salary or stipend, for a period not exceeding three months, towards defraying the expense of cleansing, papering, or painting the apartment of such master, brother, or sister.

15. One room in the hospital shall be assigned by the Governors to each brother and sister for his or her exclusive use, and every such room with its fixtures shall be maintained and kept in repair out of the income of the Charity.

Abbot's Hospital Guildford

16. The Governors shall from time to time inspect the apartments of the master, brethren, and sisters respectively, and whenever they shall consider it necessary shall direct the same to be cleansed and whitewashed, and the windows to be mended, at the expense of the occupier, and they may defray the cost by deducting the same from his or her stipend, at their discretion.

17. The Governors shall have the power of removing the master and any of the brethren or sisters, in case they shall cease to be objects of the Charity, or of immorality, insubordination, or other misconduct; provided that the removal of the master shall not be valid without the approval in writing of the Archbishop of Canterbury.

18. The master may at any time, with the concurrence of one Governor or more, suspend any brother or sister, for misconduct, from the receipt of any allowance or benefit from the Charity until the case can be reported by the master to the Governors, and decided upon by them.

19. One of the brethren shall be appointed by the Governors to be the vice-master, and during his tenure of such appointment shall receive a salary at the rate of £4 per annum, to be paid to him quarterly, in addition to his stipend as a brother. The Governors shall be at liberty at any time to remove such vice-master, at their discretion, and to appoint another in his place.

20. The oaths hitherto administered to the master, brethren, and sisters respectively shall in future be discontinued. The sisters shall also be relieved from the duty of attending the sick; and the stipend of 13*s.* 4*d.*, allowed as a remuneration for such service, and all allowances and gifts to the inmates other than those directed or provided by this scheme, shall respectively cease.

All existing regulations and usages now in with respect to the administration of the Charity, which are in any way at variance with this scheme or any of the provisions or object thereof, shall also respectively cease and be discontinued.

21. Subject to the provisions of this scheme, the Governors may from time to time prescribe such reasonable rules and regulations as they may think expedient for the government and conduct of the hospital, and the master, inmates, and officers thereof, and all rules and regulations shall be observed by the persons affected thereby.

22. If any doubt or question shall arise amongst the Governors or any of them as to the proper construction or application of any of the provisions of this scheme, or the management of the Charity, application may be made by the Governors to the Charity Commissioners for England and Wales, for their opinion and advice thereon, which opinion and advice, when given, shall be binding on the Governors and on all other persons affected thereby; and if any of the provisions hereof relating to the detailed management of the Charity, and not prescribing or defining the principal objects thereof, shall be found to be unsuitable or practically inconvenient, the same may be modified or altered or annulled by the Governors, with the sanction of the said Commissioners.

Appendix 3

23. This scheme shall be printed, and a copy given to every person who shall become a member of the governing body of the Charity, and to every master and inmate of the hospital.

Abbot's Hospital Guildford

Appendix 4

BOOK LIST

George Abbot deserves a modern, critical biography. P.A. Welsby's *George Abbot the Unwanted Archbishop 1562-1633*, London 1962, has merits in places, but is uneven, and not entirely accurate. The standard older account was A. Onslow's *The Life of Dr George Abbot, Lord Archbishop of Canterbury*, Guildford 1777. This was reprinted with additions and corrections from the article by W. Oldys in *Biographia Britannica*, London 1747, volume 1 pp 3-17. Oldys wrote to defend Abbot against Clarendon's adverse comments in *The History of the Rebellion and Civil Wars begun in the Year 1641*, Oxford 1702, volume 1.

Three shorter lives may be mentioned.

S.L. Lee in *The Dictionary of National Biography*, volume 1, where a favourable view is taken.

W.F. Hook in *Lives of the Archbishops of Canterbury*, volume 10, where a generally unfavourable view is adopted.

E. Carpenter has a judicious chapter in *Cantuar, the Archbishops in their Office*, London 1971.

The following list is not an exhaustive bibliography, or account of sources. The books and articles will provide additional information about some topics, as suggested in the notes through the book.

1. C.J. Barlow: *Archbishop Abbot's School Guildford*, Guildford 1924.
2. E. Carpenter: *Cantuar, the Archbishops in their Office*, London 1971.
3. R.A. Christophers: *George Abbot, Archbishop of Canterbury 1562-1633, A Bibliography*, Charlottesville 1966.
4. P. Collinson: *The Religion of Protestants*, Oxford 1982.
5. C. Davey: *Pioneer for Unity*, London 1987.
6. G. Davies: *The Early Stuarts 1603-1660*, Oxford 2 ed 1959.
7. P.M. Davies: *The 'Old' Royal Surrey County Hospital 1866-1980*, Guildford 1982.
8. A.C. Ducarel: 'Some Account of the Town, Church and Archiepiscopal Palace of Croydon in the County of Surrey, from its Foundation to the Year 1783' in *Bibliotheca Topographica Britannica*, London 1790, volume 2.
9. B.C. Foley:*The Eighty-five Blessed Martyrs*, London 1987.

Abbot's Hospital Guildford

10. J.K. Green: 'Some of the Schools of Guildford' in *Sidelights on Guildford History* III, Guildford 1954.

11. J.W. Headlam: 'Report on the System of Secondary Education in the County of Surrey' in *Royal Commission on Secondary Education*, London 1893, volume 7.

12. T.W. King: 'Remarks on a Brass Plate formerly in the Church of the Holy Trinity at Guildford, and now remaining in the Hospital there' in *Surrey Archaeological Collections* 1865, volume 2. (There are added copies of some Abbot wills, and extracts from Guildford registers – though not that of George Abbot's baptism at St Nicolas'. The plate is now back in Holy Trinity Church.)

13. D. Knowles and R.N. Hadcock: *Medieval Religious Houses in England and Wales*, London 1971 ed.

14. H.E. Malden: *A History of Surrey*, London cheap ed 1905 (reprinted 1977).

15. N. Malcolm: *De Dominis (1560-1624): Venetian, Anglican, Ecumenist and Relapsed Heretic*, London 1984.

16. R.B. Martin: 'Better than Ambition' in *Enter Rumour*, London 1962.

17. E. Nasalli-Rocca: 'Hospitals, History of. 1. The Christian Hospital to 1500' in *New Catholic Encyclopedia* 1967, volume 7.

18. P.G. Palmer: 'Inventory of Abbot's Hospital, Guildford, 1633' in *Surrey Archaeological Collections* 1917, volume 30.

19. P.G. Palmer (ed): *The Statutes of the Hospital of the Blessed Trinity Guildford AD 1629*, 1927.

20. W.B. Patterson: 'King James I's call for an ecumenical council' in *Councils and Assemblies* (Studies in Church History 7), Cambridge 1971.

21. D.L. Powell (compiler) and H. Jenkinson (ed): *County of Surrey, Records of Schools and Other Endowed Institutions*, Kingston 1930, volume 4.

22. B. Rackham: 'The East Window of the Chapel of Trinity Hospital, Greenwich' in *The Journal of the British Society of Master Glass-Painters* 1947-1951, volume 10.

23. S. Smith: 'Borough of Guildford' in *The Charities of the County of Surrey*, London 1839.

24. Germanos Strenopoulos: *Kyrillos Loukaris 1572-1638*, London 1951.

25. D.M. Sturley: *The Royal Grammar School Guildford*, Guildford 1980.

26. B.Taylor: *The Lower Church*, Guildford 1980.

Appendix 4

27. W. Ullmann: 'Public Welfare and Social Legislation in the Early Medieval Councils' in *Councils and Assemblies* (Studies in Church History 7), Cambridge 1971.
28. J. Walsh and B.C. Barry: *The Catholic Martyrs of England and Wales*, London 1979.
29. G.C. Williamson: *Guildford in the Olden Time*, London 1904.

Abbot's Hospital Guildford

Index

A

A. Grove & Co Ltd 108
A. Grove (Guildford) Limited 99, 107
A.H. Billimore & Son 97
Abbot, Alice 1, 14
Abbot, Anthony 1, 2, 14
Abbot, Eden 28
Abbot, George 1-34, 45, 46, 52, 53, 54, 55, 70
Abbot, John I 1, 2, 9, 50
Abbot, John II 9
Abbot, J.T. 14
Abbot, Maria 9
Abbot, Maurice I 1, 14, 24
Abbot, Morris II 1, 2, 14, 21, 23, 46, 47
Abbot, Maurice III 23, 34, 43, 46, 48, 50
Abbot, Richard I 1, 2, 22, 23, 28, 29, 33
Abbot, Richard II 31, 46
Abbot, Richard III 31
Abbot, Richard IV 31
Abbot, Robert 1, 2, 3, 4, 5, 9, 16
Abbot, Sarah 50
Abbot, Thomas I 1
Abbot, Thomas II 28
Albury 61
Alexander, Emperor of Russia 63
Alleyn, E. 20
Andrewes, L. 5, 8, 9, 10, 11
Andrewes, N. 47
Anne, Princess 112
Anne, Queen 7
Ansell, J. 64
Apted, F. 71
Archbishop Abbot's Exhibition Foundation 41, 95
Armada 6
Arminians 8
Arrowsmith, S. & E. 16
Arthur Moon and Sons 84

Astolat Company Ltd. 117
Astrete, H. 21
Athelstan, King 19
Atkinson, T. 16
Attfield, T. 60
Attorney General 37
Austen, George 21, 30
Austen, Godwin 81
Authorised Version 4, 15
Ayleworth, E. 26

B

Bacon, F. 11
Baker Exhibitions 41
Baker, T. 42
Baker, W. 21
Baker's boys 37, 39, 40
Ball, Mr. 82
Bancroft, R. 4, 5, 11, 15, 20, 28
Bannaster, W. 56
Barclays Bank 86
Barlow, W. 9
Barton, S. 51, 52
Bateman, T. 41
Beck, Miss 82
Becker, J. 97
Becket, St. Thomas 20
Beloe, H. P. 64
Benbrick, J. 53
Benson, E. W. 79, 80
Berriman, J. 45
Berry, R. 52, 53, 54, 58
Bettesworth, J. 54
Bettesworth, P. 50
Bilson, T. 5
Birch, W. 75
Bishe, Mr. 33
Bishop, W. 4, 15
Black Death 19
Blackburne, L. E. 41

Abbot's Hospital Guildford

Blacking, W.H.R. 97
Blomfield, A.W. 80
Bluett, Dr. G.M. 89, 93
Board of Agriculture and Fisheries 83
Bonner, E. 1
Book of Common Prayer 1
Book of Sports 10, 17
Boulton, W. 108
Bowle, J. 14
Bowles, H.A. 77
Boxall, J. I 64, 65, 69
Boxall, J. II 72, 73
Boyce, C.J.K. 113
Bramshill 10
Brent, M. 9
Brent, N. 9
Brewer, E. 59, 60
Brigham, R. 22, 23, 28
Brinkwell, E. 60, 61, 62
Brookes, H. 63
Brooking, C. 43
Brown, J. F. 115
Buck, J. 94
Buckeridge, J. 8, 12
Bullen, J. 84
Burchall, R. 22
Burdet, C. 57, 58
Burges, G. 23
Burkitt, H.J. 83
Burling, W.A.C. 90
Burstow Rookery farm 33, 36, 37, 38, 39, 40
Burstow parish 43, 60, 66, 67
Burt, J. 110
Butcher, R. 23
Button, Mr. and Mrs. E. 97

C

Cadwallador, R. 16
Caleb Lovejoy Foundation 93, 111
Calvinism 2, 3, 4, 8
Canterbury, Archbisop of 25, 72

Canterbury Cathedral 11
Canterbury Chapter 5
Canterbury City Council 10
Canterbury Conduit 9, 10, 17
Capital and Counties Bank 84
Carey, V. 10
Carleton, G. 16
Carling, Gill & Carling 92
Caroë, W.D. 91, 92
Caroline, Queen 63
Carr, R. 9, 16
Caryll, J. 51
Challen, G. 79, 83
Champion, J. 28, 29
Charitable Trusts Act of 1853 72, 79
Charity Commission 38, 39, 40, 41, 42, 71, 73, 74, 75, 78, 79, 82, 83, 88, 89, 90, 91, 93, 95, 96, 97, 99, 100, 102, 103, 108
Charles I, King 2, 11, 12, 13, 53, 54
Charles II, King 12, 55, 57
Charles Osenton and Company 101
Charles, Prince 12
Charlwood
   Charlwood Parish 43
   Testers (or Tifters) Farm 31, 33, 36, 37, 38, 40, 50, 60, 67
Chelsworth 1
Chiddingfold
   Brooklands Farm 27
Chitty, W. 71, 75
Christian E. 44
Christmas, G. 14
Christmas, J. 14
Christmas, M 14
Clarke, E. 55
Clarke, J. 60
Clarkes 60
Clark's College Limited 42, 44, 95, 96, 101, 107
Clemence, T.R. 87, 88, 91, 92, 96, 97, 101

Index

Clement VIII, Pope 16
Clutton, H. 37
Clutton, R. 38
Codd, L. 107
Coggan, F.D. 113, 115
Cole, W. 59, 66
College of Arms 14
College of Law 112
Colwall D. 67
Complete Art Furnisher 97
Constable family 26
Cooke, J.R. 37
Cooke, R. 40, 41
Cooper, C. 37
Corbet R. 10, 17
Corporal punishment 38
Cotton, H. 9
Court of Chancery 34, 35, 36, 68, 70, 72
Court of High Commission 6, 16
Court, S. 37
Courtnay S.H. 102
Cow and Gate 92, 107, 110, 111
Cox, W. 60
Crane, J. 29
Cranmer, T. 1, 14
Cromwell, O. 49
Cromwell, R. 49
Cromwell, T. 1
Crown Appliances Limited 108
Crown Electrical (Guildford) 114
Croydon
    10, 12, 13, 14, 20, 27, 28, 35, 52, 104
    Whitgift's Foundation 20, 21, 23, 25, 29, 72, 98, 104,

D

Dalby, R. 86
Dalman, Mrs. 82
Davenant, J. 10
Davidson, R.T. 85, 88
de Dominis, M.A. 8, 10, 16
de la Fosse, C.F. 41

Dean Hurst 44
Denham, J. 47
Dennis's motor works 92
Devereux, R. 9
Dewdney Mr. 77
Dobson, W. 23
Donellan, L. 80, 81
Dorking
    Mereden Farm 26, 27, 52, 66, 67, 71, 77, 83
    Tankerleys Farm 38, 52, 59, 66
Dort, Synod of 8
Doulton, H. 78
Dulwich
    College of God's Gift 20
Duncan, C.E. 97

E

E.C. Hughes Ltd. 114
East Grinstead, Sackville College 20
East India Company 2
Ebenezer Mears Contractors Ltd. 108
Edes, R. 15
Edwards, V 86
Edward VI, King 1, 19
Eldershaw, E. 81
Eldridge, W. 49, 66
Elizabeth I, Queen 1, 2, 6
Elizabeth II, Queen 103, 112
Elizabeth, Princess 7, 8, 13
Elizabeth, Queen 93
Elkins, R. 62, 63
Elkins, W.E. 37
Ellis, S. 87
Elsley, F.H. 85, 98
Endowed Schools Act 1869 39
English Bible 1
English Heritage 116
Ewelme
    almshouses 19
Ewhurst
    Dean Hurst Field 38

Rumbeams Farm 26, 27, 50, 60, 84, 87, 89
Salthurst Farm 38, 39, 59
Woolpits Farm 38, 58, 59, 78, 79

F

Fairbrother, P.T. 41
Farley, J. 114
Farnham Castle 47
Farnham, Urban District 42
Featley, D. 1
Felton, N. 8, 16
Fernihough, C. 41, 44
Field, T. 12
Filmer & Co 84
Filmer and Mason 80, 83
Fisher, G.F. 101, 102, 103, 109
Fisher, J. 1
Fitzgerald, M. 114
Flint, G. 57
Flutter, H. 57, 59
Flutter, P. 57, 59
Fogwill, J.W.S. 111, 113
Fogwills Ltd. 111
Ford, J. 60
Ford, L.F. 96
Franks, G.W. 90, 92
Frederic, Elector 7, 8
Frederick William III, King of Prussia 63
Frisby, F. 50
Frisby, G. 50
Fry, C. 35
Frye, G. 23
Fullagar, C. 44

G

Gabb, H.P. 94, 97
Gardiner, A.L. 98, 102
Gardiner, S. 1
Gates 73, 86, 87
Gaye, H.C. 82, 104
George I, King 7, 53
George III, King 62
George IV, King 62, 63
George V, King 81, 93
George VI, King 93
Gloyne, G.B. 110
Goad, R. 2
Goad, T. 2, 8
Godalming
  Wyatt's Almshouses 42
Godfrey, W.H. 91
Goodwin, S. 57
Goodwyn, E. 26
Goodyer, J. 53
Goodyer, Mr. 56
Goodyer, W. 57
Graham, T.W. 41
Grant, C.F. 82
Green, A.J.B. 41, 102
Greenoff, W.A. 114
Gregory XV, Pope 8
Grove, A. 95, 96, 99,
Guild of Servants of the Sanctuary 91, 103
Guildford
  Archbishop Abbot's School 36, 39, 40, 41, 43, 72, 85, 86, 96
  Bluecoat School 36, 37, 80
  Board of Guardians 35, 36
  Borough Council 41, 42, 83, 90, 95, 98, 102, 110, 113, 115, 116, 117
  Cannon Brewery 40
  Cathedral 108
  Christchurch 44
  Crown Inn 36, 38, 40, 43, 44
  Crown Tap Diocese 41
  Dominican Friary 1, 22, 67
  Grammar School 2, 20, 21, 30, 39, 43, 72, 112
  Half Moon Inn 21, 43
  Hillier House 105, 111
  Holy Trinity 25, 41, 56, 61, 77, 80, 97, 108

Index

George Abbot's tomb 14, 17, 56, 58, 63, 66, 67, 77, 80, 84, 93, 97, 98, 105
Holy Trinity, Rector of 24, 54, 72, 87
Horse and Groom 111
Mayor of 21, 23, 24, 25, 33, 34, 35, 48, 61, 62, 72, 82
Old Cloth Hall 42, 95, 101, 107, 110, 111, 112, 116
St Luke's Hospital 43
St Mary's 1
St Mary's, Rector of 24, 27
St Nicolas' 2, 16, 23, 44
St Nicolas', Rector of 24, 25, 28, 54, 72
St Saviour's, parish of 115, 116
St Saviour's with Stoke-next-Guildford 115, 116
St Thomas' Hospital
Spital 19, 20, 30
Stoke, Hospital 111
Stoke, parish of 115, 116
Stoke-next-Guildford, Rector of 72
The Half Moon 21
Thomas Baker's School 20
Three Mariners Inn 2, 14
Three Pigeons Inn 86, 98
Union Workhouse 35
Guildford Electricity Supply Company 83
Guildford Rural District Council 42, 95
Guildford Society 113
Guildford to Leatherhead railway 77
Guilford, Earl of 104
Gumm, G. 57, 59
Gumm, W. 57

H

H.P. Nott Ltd. 101
H.W. Frampton & Co. 92
Haberdashers' Company 111
Haines, G. 46

Hall, J. 12, 17
Hall Deane field 83
Hambledon 42
Hamilton, G. 5
Hamilton pf Dalzell, Lord 114
Hampton Court Conference 4
Harding, Mr. 73
Hargreaves, H.C. 102, 108
Harknett, R.P. 117
Harmer, J. 15
Harris 89
Harris, H. 80, 81, 82, 83, 84, 85
Harrison, W. 50
Harsnett, S. 13, 15, 17
Harte, W. 23
Harwood, J. 27
Harwood, J. 26
Haslemere 42
Hatchard, T.G. 72, 73, 75
Hawkedon 1
Hawkins, P. 10, 17, 21
Haydon, S. 37
Haydon, T. 37
Heath, J. 23
Heather, G. 71
Henrietta Maria, Queen 12
Henry, Prince 3, 4, 7, 11, 16
Henry, M. 9
Henry VIII, King 2, 19
Herbert, H.G. 41
Herbert, W. 11
Heseltine, M. 114
Heylin, P. 15
Hickman, Chief Officer 86
Hicks, J.B. 81
Higgins, S. 98
Higlett & Hammond 92, 97
Higlett, H.S. 41
Hill, F.F. 116
Hill, T. I 3, 4
Hill, T. II 26
Hill, W. 45

Hillar, A. 45
Hoath 12
Hocking, M.W. 108, 109
Holland, J. 48, 49, 50, 51, 52, 57
Holroyd, Captain 110
Holy Trinity Amenity Group 113
Home, G. 4, 5
Home Office 99
Hooke, A. 69, 70
Hooke, W. 70
Horne Farm 33, 40, 41, 42
Horner, H. 47, 48
Horsham
   Highlands Farm 26, 27, 30, 31, 58, 59,
     60, 63, 64, 67, 77, 83, 84, 89, 95,
     100
   Hornbrook Farm 77, 84, 89, 99
Horsley
   Railway Hotel 81
House of Commons 12
House of Lords 5
Housing Corporation 115
Howard, F. 9, 16
Howson, J. 12
Hurst, Mr. 58
Hutton, G.M. 94, 98
Hutton, L. 15
Hyde, E. 6
Hyde, P. 78

I

Ide, E. 93
Importers Retail Salerooms Ltd 114
Importers Tea Stores Limited 108
Iredell, Mrs. 65

J

Jackman, T. 35, 57, 61, 62
Jackman sisters 61, 62, 65, 69, 70
James I, King
   3, 4, 5, 6, 7, 8, 9, 10, 11, 12, 22
James II, King 51

James VI, King 4
Jeale, C. 57
Jelly, Mrs. 36
Jennings, J. 60
Johnsons 93
Juxon, W. 50

K

Kay, W. 47, 48
Kellison, M. 12
Kelly, A.L. 41
Kempe, N. 21, 30, 46
Kettle, H. 56
Keyes, C. 24, 29
King, J. 8, 9
Kingsley, W. 9, 13
Kingston-upon-Hull 2
Kirwan, E.C. 82, 88, 90, 93
Kitchiner, R.G. 23
Kritopoulos, M. 8

L

L.T. Deeprose Ltd 115
Lamb, A. 5
Lambeth Palace 8, 10, 13
   Palace Chapel 5, 9
   Palace Library 11
Lang, C.G. 90, 93
Larkins, R.H. 56
Laud, William
   3, 5, 6, 7, 8, 9, 10, 11, 12, 13, 14,
   16, 30, 45, 47
Laura Ashley Ltd 112, 116
Ledger, L. 57
Legate, B. 6
Leigh, Mr. 47
Leo XIII, Pope 14
Leslie, J.R. 114, 115, 117
Lewis, Mrs. 80
Lexiconi Restoration & Development
   Company Limited 116, 117
Lidgate, R. 37, 38

Index

Lingfield, J. 58
Local Government Act, 1972 42, 111
London
  Charthouse 20
  great fire of 51
  Hospital of King James 20
  London House 5, 12
  The Savoy 8
London to Worthing railway 77
Loseley 16, 30
Loukaris, K. 8
Lowe, T. 57
Lower, W.G. 39, 40, 80
Lowndes & Drury 87
Ludham, T. 36, 72
Lunn, H.M. 41

M

M. Avery & Sons 97
Mabanke, Mr. 59
Macfarland, J. 38, 39
Macmillan, J.V. 94
Mangles, Ross Donelly 37, 73, 104
Manners-Sutton, C. 15
Marten 9
Martin, E. 23
Martin, F.O. 71
Martin, J. 34
Martin, T. 14
Martin's Plat 44
Martyn, J. 59
Martyr, J. 57, 58
Mary, Queen 1, 14
Mary, Queen of Scots 6
Master, C.H. 40
Mawson, J. 16
Maxfield, T. 16
Merriman, H.G. 72
Merrow churchyard 62, 77, 83, 89
  Hall Place Farm 26, 27, 50, 58, 64, 67, 71, 77, 83, 84, 89, 90

Merrow, the Marsh 80
Merrow Small Farm 52, 55, 57, 59
Mervyn, Graham 111
Midland Clock Company 93
Millenary Petition 4
Ministry of Health 90
Mitchell, W. 84, 85
Mitchells Bros. 40, 44
Montague, J. 5
Montague, R. 12
Montague, Bishop 13
Montaigne, G. 8, 10, 12, 16
More, G. 16, 22, 25, 26, 28
More, T. 1
More-Molyneux, J. 73
More Molyneux, Jane 62
Morton, T. 10
Moss, John 122
Mostyn, J.W. 107, 108, 109, 111
Mostyn, Mrs 111
Moth, H. 57
Municipal Corporations Act 104
Munro, A. 63
Murray, J. 58
Murray, W. 12
Myles, Mr. 14

N

Napper, G. 16
National Assistance Board 107, 109
National Association of Almshouses 109, 114
National Fire Service 99
Nationwide Building Society 115
Nealds, J. 39
Neile, R. 5, 9, 12
Newport, R. 16
New Stone & Restoration Co. Limited 117
Newland, W. 37
Nolan, M. 62
North, F. 69

Abbot's Hospital Guildford

Nye, E. 112, 113, 114
Nye, Saunders & Partners 114

O

Oates, Miss 110
Onslow, A.P. 73
Onslow, 1st Earl 63, 78
Onslow, 2nd Earl 67
Onslow, 4th Earl 40
Onslow 47
Overall, J. 8
Overton, W. 5
Owen, J. 17
Oxford University 3, 4, 8, 11, 14
   Broadgates Hall 11
   Balliol College 3, 4, 8, 9, 11
   Corpus Christie College 31
   Merton College 9
   Pembroke College 11
   Queen's College 65
   St John's College 3
   St Mary's 3
   University College 3, 5, 11

P

Palmer, J. 72, 73
Palmer, P.G. 39, 43, 85, 86, 88, 89, 90, 91, 92
Pardye, R. 23
Parker, Margaret 30
Parker, Matthew 2
Parkhurst, J. 16
Parkhurst, T. 35
Parsons, James 50
Parsons, John 50
Passmore, H. 96
Paulet, E. 16
Paynter, S. 36
Peake, G.H. 94
Pearce, J. 37
Pearson, C.C. 102
Pearson, W.H. 36

Pell, E. 56
Percival, R. 48
Percy, F.H.G. 104
Percy, R.H. 98, 100, 103, 107, 108, 109, 110, 111, 113, 115
Perin, J. 4
Perkins, W. 4, 15
Piggott, W. 70
Pigott, S. 53
Pilcher, H.D. 93, 94
Pimm, J. 72
Piper, H. 72, 73
Polesden, T. 33
Pontefract, St Nicholas' Hospital 29
Poor Law Amendment Act of 1834 35
Porter, R. 80
Porter, R.F.H. 108
Portsmouth, A. 83, 85
Potter, H. 63
Powell, A. 53
Powell, L. 97, 102
Poyle estate 30, 43, 48
Price, J. 60
Privy Council 6, 7, 13
Purse, R. 21
Puttock, A. 81, 107
Pyke, J. 94

R

R. Holford 108
R. Porter & Co. Ltd. 103
R. Wood and Son 92
Ramsey, A.M. 109, 115
Rapkins, J.B. 90
Rapley, Joan 23
Rapley, John 23
Ravens, R. 15
Ravis, Thomas, Bishop of London 5
Reading School 3
Redfern, H. 87, 88
Richards, J. 73
Roberts, J. 16

Roberts, T. 56
Robinson, S. 35, 64
Roman Catholicism 2, 4, 6, 7, 8, 8, 12, 13
Rouse, Mr. 38
Rule, Mrs. 81
Runcie, R.A.K. 115
Russell, G. 36, 70, 71, 72
Russell, J. 61
Russell, S. 63, 64, 70
Russell, W. I 70
Russell, W. II 73

S

Sackville, R. 26
Sackville, T., Earl of Dorset 3, 4, 14, 20
Salsburys 83
Sancroft, W. 51
Sandeman, B. 77
Sanders, W.S. 80
Sands, T. 54, 55, 66
Saunders, A.E.F. 114, 115
Savile, H. 15
Saxey, W. 2
Saye, C. 50
Saye, R. 50
Scotcher, R. 34
Scotland, Church of 4, 5, 15
Scott Brownrigg & Turner 105
Scott, J.M. 114
Scott, J. 51, 66
Scott, R.D. 101, 104, 107, 109
Scott, W. 16
Scottish Parliament 110
Seaman, J. 23
Searle, J. 58
Secker, T. 58
Sells, C.J. 78, 89
Sells, T.J. 72, 73, 75, 78
Send Meadow 90
Sex & Son 109
Shaw, J. 51

Shaw, S. 51
Shaw-Lefevre, G. 72, 73
Shawcross, W. 87, 88
Sheldon, G. 15, 50, 51
Shepherd, R. 72
Sheppard, W.G.L. 102
Shillingford, Mr. 73
Shore, P. 114
Sibthorpe, R. 12
Simmonds, W. 40
Sinclair, R.S.B 102
Sizer, S.R. 116
Slater, A. 39, 40
Smallpeice and Merriman 98, 110
Smallpeice, H.P. 78, 83
Smallpeice, Job 38
Smallpeice, John 53
Smallpeice, M 70, 73, 74, 78, 82, 83
Smallpeice, T. I 53, 54, 55
Smallpeice, T. II 73
Smallpeice, W.H. & M. 73
Smallpeice, W. 47
Smith, E. 52
Smith, H. 65
Smith, S.H. 102
Smith, T. 47
Smith, W. and T. 76, 77
Smith, W. 72, 73
Smither, J. 61
Smither, S. 61
Smithfield
   St Bartholomew's Hospital 19
Snelling, H. 34, 46, 47
Somers, T. 16
Somerset, Duke of 1
South Kensington Museum 76
Southam, E.G. 94, 102
Southerne, W. 16
Spain 7, 8, 10, 11
Spenser, E. 17
Spottiswoode, J. 5
St Catherine's Woodlands 27, 28

Abbot's Hospital Guildford

St John's Ambulance Corps 85, 86
Stanley Ellis Ltd 96
Stanton, J. 34
Star and Garter Homes 111, 112
Stedman, J. 37
Stevens, G. 9, 66, 108
Stevens, J. 54
Stillington
    West Wantley Farm 27, 46, 51, 78, 83
Story, J. 1, 14
Stoughton, Shepherd's Farm 78, 83, 89, 90, 95
Stoughton, H. 56, 57
Stow-on-the-Wold, Holy Trinity Hospital 29
Strudwick, G. 39
Strudwick, Mr. 73
Suffolk
    Earl of 6, 9
Suffragettes 81
Sumner, J.B. 37, 70, 73
Sumpster, J.M. 41
Surrey Advertiser 76, 79, 111, 112, 113
Surrey County Council 41, 42, 95, 110, 111
Surrey Fire Officer 58
Surrey Historic Buildings Trust Ltd. 117
Surrey Times 79
Sutton, B. 22
Sutton, T. 20
Swayne, G.O. 107, 115
Swayne, T.G. 41
Sydserf, T. 15

T

Tanzania 122
Taunton, T. 40
Taverner, W.S. 88
Taylor, B. 113
Taylor, E. 113, 116
Taylor, F. 2
Taylor, H.G. 113, 116, 117

Taylor, W. 70
Tegge, J. 24
Tenison, T. 52
Teck, Princess Mary of ??
Terry, R. 23
Terry, T. I 53
Terry, T. II 73, 78, 79, 83
Teulon, S.S. 44
The Black Book 69
The Edinburgh Woollen Mill Ltd. 116
The Extraordinary Black Book 69
The Charities in the County of Surrey 69
The Mark of Merrow 80
The Times 111, 113
The West Surrey Times 79, 80
Thomson, G. 15
Thornborough, G. 49
Thules, J. 16
Tidy, W. 70, 75
Tillotson, E. 30
Tisdale, T. 11
Tower, F.E. 75, 79
Town and Country Planning Act 114
Townsend, A. 60
Townsend, T. 60
Townson, R. 16
Trasey, S. 56
Tribe & Robinson 88
Tribe, R.H. 97
Triggs Turner 95, 98, 114
Trimmer, R.W. 75
Tunstall, T. 16

U

University of Surrey 112
Upton, J. 60
Upton, T. 60
Urban VIII, Pope 8

V

Valpy, A.S. 79, 80, 81
van Prizzn, A. 49

168

van Somer, P. 46
Vernon, E. 54
Victoria, Queen 79, 81
Villiers, G. 7, 8, 11, 12, 13
Virginia Company 2

W

Wake, W. 54, 57
Wale, E.G.R. 91, 92, 93, 98, 103
Wall, T. 47
Wallis, M. 57, 58, 59
Wantley 74
Warnham, W. 15
Warwick, J. 57
Waverley Borough Council 42
Weale, J. 37
Wells, Mrs. 82
Weston, R. 34
West Surrey Times 78
Wey Navigation 34
White, F. 12
White, G.L. 59, 60
Whitgift, J. 20, 21, 24, 27, 30
Whitgift, R. 20
Whittaker, D. 97
Wicks, D. 56
Wightman, E. 6
Wightwick, R. 11
Wilkins, D. 103, 107
Williams, A. 102
Williams, J. 10, 11
Williamson, J. 89
Wilson, G.S. 97
Wiltshier Ltd. (Reading) 114
Winchester
  Bishop of 25, 81
  Cathedral 3, 5, 11
  St Cross Hospital 19, 69, 104
Windsor
  St George's Chapel 8
Wink, E. 115
Wink, M. 115

Wonham, J. 50
Wood, A. 1
Wood, E. 55, 56
Woodward, M. 53
Woodyer, H. 76, 77, 80, 87
Woodyer, R. 40
Woolley, J. 59, 60
Worcester
  All Saints' 2
  St Oswald's Hospital 19
Wrenno, R. 16
Wright, J. 23
Wrist, C. 81
WVS 100
Wyatt, R. 20

Y

Yardley, J. 29, 33, 34, 45, 46
York, St Peter's Hospital 19, 29
York, Duke of 81
York House Conference 12
Young Men's Christian Association 42

Z

Zouche, Lord 10